ANGEL BABIES

Messages from Miscarried
and
Other Lost Babies

Patricia Seaver McGivern

iUniverse, Inc.
New York   Bloomington

iUniverse books may be ordered through booksellers or by contacting:

iUniverse
1663 Liberty Drive
Bloomington, IN 47403
www.iuniverse.com
1-800-Authors (1-800-288-4677)

Because of the dynamic nature of the Internet, any Web addresses or links contained in this book may have changed since publication and may no longer be valid. The views expressed in this work are solely those of the author and do not necessarily reflect the views of the publisher, and the publisher hereby disclaims any responsibility for them.

ISBN: 978-0-595-53542-2 (sc)
ISBN: 978-1-4401-2522-5 (hc)
ISBN: 978-0-595-63610-5 (ebook)

Library of Congress Control Number: 2009925363

Printed in the United States of America

iUniverse rev. date: 04/17/2009

In loving memory of

Dillon, my angel baby.
Thank you for coming.

Harlan, my father,
W ho though on the other side, continues to give me incredible
soul gifts.

and

Patricia, my mother,
who is closer than I ever realized.

For Kylie and Meghan,

my Earth angels,

and

Tim, my love and father of all my angels,

and for

everyone who's ever lost a baby.

As the baby entered the world, it was said,
"It is important that you learn from these people you choose as
your parents,
but they should also learn from you."

And the wise soul replied,
"Yes, I have much to teach them."

"Wise Little Soul" by Hyla Molander

Contents

Acknowledgments

I extend special thanks to Gloria Aukland, who came into my life as an answer to a prayer and became my editor, mentor, and friend.

With deep gratitude, I also thank those people who have been placed in my life at exactly the right time to support, encourage, or nudge me along: Victor Borak, MD, who helped me understand my fear of writing and release it; Linda Bialow, who proofread *Angel Babies* and became a believer; Susan Carey, who stretched enough to hear me; Alice Cockrell, who has always believed me and believed in me; Beverly Coe, who encouraged me to write for the mothers who'd lost babies; Theresa Danna, who helped me find others who'd had experiences similar to mine; Barbara Gaskill, who proofread my manuscript and became my "publicity agent"; Elisabeth Hallet, who assisted with my research; Carolene Heart, who helped me understand Dillon; Maryanne Lane, who related Dillon's messages to me; Dr. Raymond Moody, whose kind words touched my heart; and the mediums who helped me to believe: Don McIntosh, J. Kenn Coulter, Gail Rhoads, John Rogers, Christine Riley, and Yvonne M. Gangone, as well as George Anderson and Andrew Barone.

Most important, I thank all those who shared their touching stories of communication with their lost babies: Mary and baby Ravine; Sarah, Anders, and baby Emilie; Debbie and baby boy; Phaedra, baby girl, and baby Jeremiah; Lee and baby Kyler; Lisa and baby Walter; Gwen and baby boy; Phyllis and friend's baby boy and girl; Holly and baby boy; Judith and baby Adam; Erin and baby Sarrah; Jane and baby boy; Sylvia and baby girl; Melissa Anne and baby Helem; Ann-Marie and baby Micah; Nadine and baby; Ellen and baby Ariella; Daniel and babies Jesse, Samuel, Brian, and Sarah; Tracey and baby girl; Kelly and baby Avery; Chris and grandmother's baby girl; Cina and baby Michael; Natalie and baby Darien; Stacey and baby Colestine; Maria and baby Leonor; Annette and baby; Nellie and baby boy; Karen and baby James; Jennifer and baby Monica; Sunny, baby Carmen and Guide Eli; Cheryl and baby; Carla and baby Isobella; Mutsumi and babies Chie and Ai.

Special thanks to Hyla Molander for permission to use her poem "Wise Little Soul."

Preface

On awaking that sunny spring day in 1995, I had no way of knowing that the course of my life would change in one pivotal moment. Had anyone suggested that my path would lead me to where I am today—working as a hypnotist specializing in past-life regression and the author of a book about spirit communication with early loss babies—I would have vehemently shaken my head in disbelief. No, I was a stay-at-home mother of two young children following a seventeen-year career in the corporate world, not a sharer of deeper truths. Or so I thought. But that day, I heard from my miscarried baby.

How could I have known before then that one of my greatest gifts lay not in carrying my baby but in learning more through his death than through his birth? His loss would cause me, both willingly and unwillingly, to stretch and grow my spiritual beliefs.

I struggled with believing that the experiences I had of my baby communicating were real and not a figment of my imagination or a sign of my impending insanity. In the moment, the communication seemed so real, but later, as a curtain seemed to close and my conscious, thinking mind activated again, the skeptic in me would return and I would question it.

To find some validation, I began to research parents and others who might have experienced such communication, and I found quite a number. Those who have contributed their personal stories to this book have shown great courage. All of the experiences are true, based on the memories of those telling their stories. Only their names have been changed, when requested, to protect their privacy. My hope and theirs is that others will come to know they are not alone in their feelings or experiences. We hope they may take comfort in knowing that we remain bonded to our lost babies through love and that life is indeed continuous.

In the first section of this book, I tell my story and how I began my research. The second section contains the results of my research: the personal stories of those who've had similar experiences. Those experiences are organized by how the communication was received, such as through dreams, hypnosis, visions, coincidences, near-death or psychic experiences, or mediation.

When I finished writing the book, I asked a friend to read it. She in turn gave it to a friend of hers to read. That friend called to tell me she was reading it as a favor since her religious beliefs were not in accord with the book's content. I swallowed hard and waited for the criticism. Several days later, she called and said two simple words: "I believe." As I began to tell people about the book, I'd often see their eyes well with tears as they all related a similar message: others need to hear this.

My hope is that this book helps heal those who've lost a baby, validates those who've had their own special experiences, enlightens those who haven't, and opens doors for anyone on the greater path of understanding the soul.

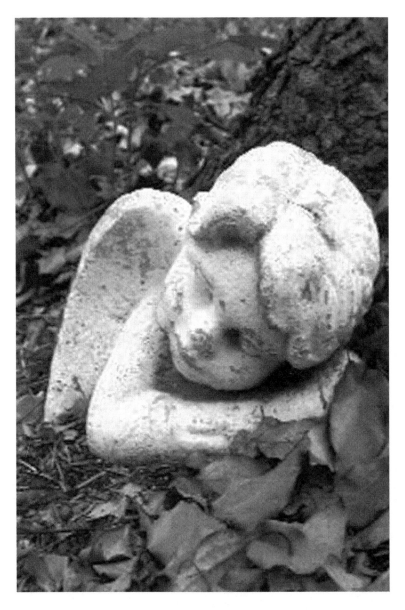

Photo by Kylie McGivern

Hearing from an Angel Baby:
I'm Right Here. I'm Right Here!

I loved the quietness of our home when my six-year-old, Kylie, was at school and my busy three-year-old daughter, Meghan, napped. Although a rare indulgence for me, I'd manage to squeeze in a nap myself on some days. So it was on that day years ago.

I was slowly waking up from napping, in that in-between state, when I heard an urgent and excited child's voice next to me exclaim, "I'm right here! I'm right *here!*" My eyes flew open, and my body jolted to a tingly full alertness. From the tone of the small voice, I had the feeling I was in trouble for getting caught lying down on the job. I turned my head in the direction of the voice. I expected to see Meghan beside my bed, near my head, but found I was alone in the room.

Puzzled by why her voice sounded so close to me when she wasn't there, I thought she must be out in the hallway, behind the closed bedroom door. "Meghan?" I called out to her. "Mommy's right here, honey," I assured her. I imagined her sitting in the hallway, propped against the door, still half-asleep, holding her blanket.

Still lying on the bed, I called, "Come to Mommy, sweetheart," waiting for her to come and snuggle with me. Again she didn't answer. Why hadn't she opened the door and come to me as she usually did? Why did her voice sound so close when she wasn't even in the same room? I waited.

"Meghan, Mommy is right here, honey," I said, hoping to coax her toward me. Resolved that she wasn't moving until I did, I went to the bathroom and splashed water on my face.

"Meghan?" I called out again. Silence filled the house. For someone who sounded so exasperated trying to let me know she was right here, why wasn't she answering me? It was unlike her not to come to me. I dried my face and peeked around the doorway. Meghan wasn't in the hallway or within sight.

Where could she be? I hadn't heard her familiar little footsteps patter off anywhere. In fact, I hadn't heard her say anything after she most assuredly let me know she was up and I wasn't. I quickly looked for her in the living room and kitchen as I became more puzzled over her whereabouts.

"Where in the world did she go?" I asked aloud as I stood completely still. The answer immediately popped into my head. *Meghan is still asleep upstairs.* I knew the words hadn't originated with me.

The hair on the back of my neck stood up, and goose bumps covered my arms. I knew with certainty that I had heard her little child's voice right next to me in the bedroom. How could she still be asleep upstairs? I bolted up the stairs, taking them two at a time. As I turned the corner to look into her bedroom I found her in a deep sleep, sprawled on her pink princess bed.

I stood almost paralyzed as I tried to discern how I could have heard her voice next to me when she was upstairs asleep. Neither the radio nor the television was turned on, and no one else was in the house. I paused, trying to assimilate the information and dissect what I'd heard. The voice was clear and insistent—and exasperated—almost as though I were a complete idiot for not noticing the obvious. *If it wasn't Meghan I heard,* I asked myself, *just who had been calling?*

As quickly as I asked the question, I heard the answer in my mind. *It wasn't Meghan's voice you heard. It was the baby you lost.* Every hair on my body stood on end as I stared at Meghan's sleeping form. I sucked in a short breath. The answer did not come from me. My eyes slowly moved from Meghan to the image of me in the hallway mirror. I swallowed hard.

"What?" I murmured, stunned at the possibility. I ran down the hall to my bedroom and sat on the loveseat at the foot of my bed. Goose bumps now covered my body from head to toe as I quickly blurted out, "I know it's you, my baby. Please come and show yourself to me."

I acted on impulse alone. I didn't stop to think that what I was saying might be irrational. I quickly reasoned that if I could hear a voice, then maybe I could see my child. I wanted more. I wanted to *see* the baby.

With my eyes open as big as saucers and my mouth agape, I sat motionless, holding my breath and staring intently at the space in front of me, waiting for the unthinkable to happen—for the baby to appear. Each second felt like an eternity as my heart pounded wildly.

Frozen to the chair, I tried to make sense of what had just happened. Even though I hadn't been fully awake, I knew I wasn't asleep or dreaming. I knew with certainty I had heard a voice that sounded as if it were right next to me. It was a little voice, a small child's voice, and by the no-nonsense tone, the child was rather impatient with my inability to see the obvious. The inflection of the voice seemed to say, "If you'd just open your eyes, you'd see me!" I repeated the words, mimicking their tone, "I'm right here, I'm right *here!*" Was it really possible that I had just heard the baby I had lost?

The magnitude of my experience began to sink in, and as it did, I began to think about the baby I'd miscarried. Why had he or she come to me now? Was there something special about the day? It was April 26. The baby had been due May 1, four years earlier. Was it possible the baby was telling me when it would have been born? I wasn't certain, and it didn't matter. That the baby had come and I'd heard its voice was incredible enough. The baby's words echoed in my mind throughout the day. I could hardly wait to tell my husband, Tim, when he arrived home that evening.

Tim and I had met in college. I was at ease being with him even on the first night we met, and we talked into the wee hours of the morning. I knew that night he would become someone special in my life. We had made that kind of connection.

Tim had barely walked through the door when I told him excitedly, "You aren't going to believe what happened today." I pulled him by the hand to the sofa. The sofa was reserved for our serious conversations, and I wanted his complete attention.

I took his hand and held it in mine. "When I put Meghan down for a nap today," I began, "I decided to take a nap myself and lay down in the downstairs bedroom because it's quieter there." Enthusiastically, I told

Tim about my experience, finishing with a deep sigh. "Can you believe it? I heard our baby," I gushed.

Looking intently at me, Tim saw my excitement. Tenderly, he held me and replied, "That *is* incredible." We sat locked in each other's arms, silent with our own thoughts. Although it stretched his belief system, I knew he believed me.

During the following week, my mind repeatedly replayed those few brief moments of hearing the baby's voice. I yearned for a physical connection to the baby, and so I climbed into the attic and pulled out a shoebox containing all the reminders of my lost little one and took it to the bedroom. Lovingly, I took each memento from the cardboard box, holding each item so delicately, as though it were a sacred treasure.

The first treasure was a plastic home pregnancy test I had used to find out whether I was pregnant. The positive sign still showed. It was the only physical proof I had that our baby had existed. I caressed the plastic case softly before gently placing it to my side.

Next, I took out the stack of condolence cards we had received and began reading them. Many seemed to understand the depth of our grief, and their personal notes touched me. As I read each card, my heart became heavier and heavier. The painful loss of our baby more than four years earlier came rushing back. I was unable to hold the pain inside any longer. Tears began falling silently, slowly sliding down my cheeks before spilling onto my lap, tears that weren't satisfied until accompanied by heartbreaking sobs. They flowed from a place deep within me, a place I thought I had healed.

I was surprised at the depth of my sorrow since, after the miscarriage, I had worked through the grieving process in various therapeutic settings. In one group setting, we had role-played a baptism and funeral for the baby. When asked what the baby's name was, Tim and I just looked at each other with a blank stare. We hadn't known the sex of the baby, and our intuitive feelings were not in agreement. I felt the baby was a boy, and Tim was just as certain it was a girl. So we had never named the baby. The person role-playing the religious figure saw our perplexed look and asked, "What if we name the baby Angel?" I loved the name so much that I burst into tears as I held an empty, worn blanket, imagining our baby was somewhere inside its folds.

As much as I liked the name Angel, it was as though we had consciously forgotten it because whenever we talked about the miscarriage, we continued to refer to our child as "the baby."

Would I ever be able to think about the baby without crying? I wondered. Was my only connection with the baby one of pain and loss?

As I calmed my grief, I realized that there could be no pain without love. The love had come first. The love was real. "The love survived," I whispered with a deep sigh, "even though the baby didn't."

I placed the items lovingly back into the shoebox and replaced the lid. "I just wish I knew the sex of the baby," I muttered before putting the box away.

That evening, I awoke in the middle of the night to a soft voice at the foot of my bed gently saying, "Mommy?" I bolted upright in bed to see which of my two children needed me. I looked to where I'd heard the voice, but no one was there. I couldn't see either of my girls. "Meghan?" I softly called out. "Kylie?" Neither child answered. I looked at my sleeping husband to see whether the voice had awakened him, but he seemed undisturbed. A deep sleeper, I was always amazed at how my maternal alarm went off when I heard one of my children.

I got out of bed and searched the bedroom floor for them, softly calling out their names again before noticing our bedroom door was still closed. Instantly, I realized they couldn't have been in our bedroom because they would never close the door behind themselves. Besides, it was usually the door opening that would awaken me before they spoke. The voice I heard was soft and gentle and in my bedroom. Goose bumps rushed over my skin as I realized the voice I heard wasn't either of my girls. It was the baby—again.

Just to be sure, I walked down the hall to the girls' bedroom, opened the door, and found them cozily tucked in and sleeping soundly. "Mommy's here. Do you need anything?" I asked. Neither child responded.

Walking back to our bedroom, I said aloud but softly, "I heard you, darling baby. I know it was you," thinking it might be important to acknowledge what I'd heard.

As soon as the alarm went off the next morning, I nudged Tim awake. "Honey, did you hear either of the girls last night?

"No," he answered sleepily.

"You didn't hear someone say, 'Mommy?'" I questioned.

"No," he answered quickly.

"Well did you hear me get up?" I asked.

"No," he responded as he rolled over.

"Last night I heard a child's voice say 'Mommy?' It even woke me up. It couldn't have been the girls because our bedroom door was closed," I explained to him, "And so was theirs," I added. But I was the one needing an explanation. "Tim, it was the baby again."

A deeper part of me seemed to accept fully what I had heard, but a more rational part of me knew that hearing from our baby was, well, perhaps abnormal. "Am I going crazy?" I asked Tim, thinking I should rule that out as well. After all, he was a licensed mental health counselor. Surely he would know if I were losing my sanity.

"No, honey," he replied earnestly, although I wondered whether he was just being kind.

I replayed the sound of the little voice in my mind as I got dressed. My day was starting with a massage, which was an irregular indulgence I enjoyed. Maryanne, my massage therapist, was excellent, and I was fascinated with her office. She was interested in the metaphysical, and although I wasn't really sure what that meant, I was intrigued. To the side of her lobby was a room where she sold incense, crystals, and books. I was always curious about the items she had and wandered around the room with only one thought in mind: *Who buys this stuff?*

Maryanne had once told me her office was like a beacon for people, and it was interesting to see who walked through her door. I certainly wondered how I had ended up there, but as foreign as her office seemed to me, it also felt very safe.

In her massage room, there was a large framed picture of a Native American man. When I questioned her about it, she said she had seen her spirit guide while in meditation, and the picture reminded her of that guide. I was fascinated.

We would usually talk for a few minutes before she began massaging me, and then we'd both remain quiet for the rest of the massage. Having two young children, I relished the silence.

What I liked most was that halfway through the massage, when she turned me over to massage my back, I began having conversations in my mind with my parents—my dead parents. Relaxed and quiet, I would simply begin by imagining I was at a home Tim and I had rented in Jamaica soon after the miscarriage. I'd be out on the pool deck, relaxing on a chaise lounge as I'd wait for my parents to come. The doors were always open in that house, enabling me to look through the back doors, the living room, and the front doors, to the front yard. The first time my parents appeared, they were in the living room. The light from the opened front doors behind them caused them to appear as darkened silhouettes. A cocoon of bright light surrounded their bodies. As they walked toward me, through the open back doors and into the sunlight, I could see them clearly in human form, the halo of white light gone.

I assumed I was making it up, even though it seemed far beyond my imaginative capability. It was so wonderful to see my parents again that I allowed myself to have the fantasy. I reasoned that I must be very good at it, because I could actually feel the softness of their hands as they held mine. They looked slightly younger than they were when they died, and more important, they were healthy again. In this state of relaxation and imagination, my parents and I had conversations.

Because their advice was so different from what I would have wanted to hear, I began to question whether I was imagining seeing them in my mind or if they were somehow real.

Some of my talks with my parents were more powerful than others, but most were highly emotional, and I was moved enough to cry. Whatever the visits were, I found great comfort in them and felt as though I had actually been with them.

If Maryanne could see her spirit guide with her eyes wide open, I knew she was someone I could share my experiences with and not be judged crazy. Still, I chose not to tell her. Perhaps just knowing I could be with my parents and feel safe was good enough.

When I walked into Maryanne's office that morning, she welcomed me with her warm and friendly smile and ushered me to her private massage room to undress and lie on my back. As she began massaging me, she asked in her usual upbeat tone, "What's up?" I looked intently at her and knew she wouldn't think I was completely mad if I told her about hearing the baby. After all, I reasoned to myself, I only hear voices, but she sees dead people.

"I've been thinking a lot about a baby I lost," I said quietly. Maryanne continued massaging me. Silence filled the small room as my thoughts wandered to the events of the week.

"He's here," she said calmly. Startled, I quickly opened my eyes, looking to be sure I was properly covered. If a man were present, I wanted some privacy. Maryanne was looking through the open door to her office.

Wondering who was out of my view I asked, "Who's here?" as I continued adjusting the sheets.

"Your son is here," she replied as she continued looking straight ahead to nothingness.

"*Who's* here?" I asked, certain I had misunderstood her.

"Your son is here," she repeated.

I looked again in the direction she was looking, through the open door, but no one was there, at least no one I could see. A thousand thoughts and questions instantly flooded my brain.

"My baby is a boy?" I asked, amazed she was able to see something I couldn't. I always felt the baby would be a boy, but I had never mentioned that to her.

"What does he look like?" I blurted out. "Please describe him to me."

"He's a towhead," she said with a surprised tone, smiling. "He has really blonde hair. And he has big blue eyes," she declared.

"How old is he?" I asked, wanting more validation and knowing I had not divulged how long it had been since the miscarriage.

"I'm not good at telling ages," she answered somewhat apologetically, as though she would disappoint me by her answer. My heart dropped. "But he looks to be four years old," she replied.

My heart skipped a beat. She was right. He would have been four had he been born. Excited at the possibility she was really seeing my baby, I implored her to tell me more.

"He's wearing a red shirt and denim overalls, and he has one of those red wagons. He's saying, 'I'm a'truckin.'" The skeptic in me analyzed her description, silently questioning its truth, yet I knew I probably would have dressed him in little overalls.

"He has a bear in the wagon. It's a small, brown, woolly bear. Not like the new ones. It's the way bears used to look years ago," she continued. She described perfectly an antique-looking bear I had been attracted to in a craft store. I was so drawn to it that I bought it, not for either of the children, but for me. I had never bought myself a stuffed toy, and I felt a little embarrassed when I did. I couldn't explain, even to myself, why I had to have that bear, but I recalled my excitement as I purchased it.

I couldn't believe I was now hearing Maryanne describe what sounded like the same bear.

"What's my son's name?" I asked.

"He's telling me it's a name Tim thought of," she replied, continuing to stare at the same midair space through the door. I ignored her reference to Tim's names and rattled off all the names I had wanted, certain it was one of them.

"No," she said with a lilt to her voice, gently correcting me, "he's saying it's a name *Tim* chose."

How did she know those weren't names Tim chose? Miffed it wasn't one of the names I wanted, I attempted to remember names Tim liked, but I couldn't remember any. How in the world was I supposed to remember a name Tim suggested nearly five years earlier? I threw out the name Ryan and several others I liked and then drew a blank. Just as I was about to give up a name suddenly popped in my mind. "Dillon?" I asked, unsure.

Dillon is an Irish Gaelic name meaning loyal or faithful, and it was the very first name Tim had suggested.

"Yes," she said, "he's telling me his name is Dillon." A rush of excitement filled me.

"Flip me over," I instructed her. "I want to talk to him myself." If I could speak to my parents in this manner, I reasoned, maybe I could speak to my son this way, too.

I turned on my stomach, closed my eyes, and took a deep breath. As I exhaled, I silently began calling out to him in a singsong voice. "Dillon, Dillon, it's Mommy. I'm here. I love you. I miss you." As the emotion of the moment filled my eyes with tears, I told him silently, "I love you so much, Dillon."

Suddenly, I felt him behind my left shoulder. He was so close to me. I couldn't see him, but I could feel his presence. Afraid our time together was limited and not sure how much he'd heard of what I'd already said, I couldn't get the words out quick enough, "I love you, Dillon. I've missed you so very much." In my mind, I hurled the words out to him.

Sweetly, softly, I heard his reply, "I know, Mommy." It was the same little voice I had heard before. "I love you, too," he said.

My brain felt overloaded. There were so many things I wanted to say to him that I couldn't form a single coherent thought fast enough before I heard another voice, an adult male, and I felt it had come from in front of me and to my right, although I couldn't see anyone. "What about Meghan?" the older male voice asked.

"Who is that?" I questioned. "Who else is here?" I knew the voice hadn't come from Dillon or me, and I was very annoyed someone else would barge in at this particular time. After all, I sputtered in my mind, I was talking to my miscarried baby. "What does Meghan have to do with Dillon?" I screamed in frustration.

Dillon, to my surprise, answered the question. "Meghan was supposed to have come with me before. I fulfilled my mission, but she wanted you to be her Mommy so much that she chose to come back to you."

"What?" I was shocked utterly speechless with this information. "She what?" I questioned silently. "I was pregnant with twins?" My mind drifted off to analyze the information. Could it be possible? I remembered reading stories about women who didn't discover they were pregnant with twins until late in their pregnancy, but …

My mind raced to the day of the miscarriage and a comment my doctor had made to me after I had asked her why I was hemorrhaging. "It's as though there's a tear, and the baby is holding on," she explained. I found her words comforting. I liked the idea that the baby didn't want to leave any more than I wanted him or her to go, but I always thought it was one baby. Could the baby who was holding on have been Meghan and not Dillon? I returned to my inner mind and sensed Dillon and the other presence were gone.

Maryanne continued massaging me quietly as I mulled over everything in my mind, not wanting to break the spell by talking. I quietly dissected the conversation I'd just had with Dillon.

For a few minutes, my mind felt bombarded and my senses flooded. Had I imagined the whole thing? No, I answered firmly. This was far beyond anything I could have imagined.

The massage over, Maryanne left the room while I lay still for a few moments, attempting to process everything that had occurred. I got dressed and shuffled out to the lobby, half dazed.

Maryanne acted so casually about what had just happened that I assumed she must see spirits all the time.

"That was incredible," I mumbled, still dazed.

"When I first saw him," Maryanne began, "he told me, 'That's my mommy on the table. She wanted to know what sex I was.' And his coloring was so surprising," she added. You and Tim both have dark hair, and so I couldn't believe how blonde this kid was. And his big blue eyes! What color are Tim's eyes?"

"Green," I answered.

"What color are yours?" she said, looking at me, trying to figure it out.

"Blue, but they usually look gray and sometimes even green."

"What color hair and eyes do your girls have?"

"Blonde hair, Meghan especially so. Both have big blue eyes," I answered her as her mouth dropped open. Maryanne could not have known that, never having seen our daughters or even a photo of them. I knew without question she had described our son.

Maryanne's next client arrived, and our conversation ended. I walked out of her office, made my way to my car, and fell into the driver's seat. Too immobilized to drive, I sat very still and thought about Dillon, my son. As the shock wore off, excitement began to flood my senses. I couldn't wait to get home and tell Tim.

As I drove into our garage, I honked the car horn to alert Tim I was home. Running upstairs, I began calling, "Tim, Tim!" I opened the kitchen door and found him sitting in our rocking chair, reading the newspaper.

"I have something incredible to tell you," I began in an excited voice. Tim sat quietly as I recounted my experience with Maryanne and Dillon. I ended my story by asking, "Can you believe it?" Tim looked at me expressionless, not saying a word. Was he trying to form a sentence? Was he considering psychiatric care for me?

As I waited for him to respond, Meghan came running to greet me. I picked her up for her usual hug and kiss, looked deeply into her eyes, and told her, "I'm so glad I'm your mommy." I looked over to Tim, who had gone back to reading the paper, and felt disappointed by his lack of interest in the amazing events that had happened. Granted, it was difficult for him to believe, but it was unlike him not to say something, not even to ask a question. His response was a blank stare as though he hadn't heard a word I had said. I walked to the living room, holding Meghan, and mulled over Tim's lack of response. Did he not believe me?

This experience was different from my experience of hearing the baby's voice. This one involved another person saying she saw and heard things, which opened up the question of her credibility. What if I had imagined the conversation with Dillon in my head to fill a need within me?

"Tim's right," I muttered to Meghan as we sat down on the floor to play. "It's impossible." My last thought about Dillon and the events of that day ended on a note of disbelief.

I can't explain what I myself don't fully understand. Maybe his communication was just too big for me to internalize. I can't help but wonder what would have happened if I had never returned to see Maryanne two months later.

Dillon's Message

"So what did Tim think of our last session?" Maryanne asked politely as she adjusted the sheets over my body before beginning the massage.

It had been nine weeks since my last massage. She wanted me to remember it, but I had let disbelief cloud my memory. Since I couldn't recall it, I was fishing for a reply. "Did I enjoy the massage?" I asked, wondering if I had correctly guessed the answer she was looking for.

Maryanne looked at me strangely and tilted her head slightly as she replied, "No, what did Tim think of the session?"

Perplexed and frustrated that I seemed to be missing the point, I asked, "What do you mean?"

Looking at me almost sternly, she asked, "What did he think of my seeing the baby you lost?"

I bolted upright. "What?" I blurted out. For a split second, I had no idea what she was talking about. Shocked, I quickly scanned my memory of my last massage with her, and in a sudden flash, the memory flooded my mind.

"Oh my God!" I exclaimed. "How could I forget?" I looked at her for an explanation. Forgetting something so meaningful wasn't something I'd ordinarily do. Hurriedly, I chastised myself.

Maryanne looked at me, appearing rather incredulous, and asked, "What was his name again?"

My mind went blank. Feeling as though I'd failed my child in the most catastrophic way, tears filled my eyes as I whispered in shock, "I don't remember." I tried as hard as I could to remember his name, not believing I could forget something so sacred. "How could I forget?" I repeated, hoping Maryanne would provide an answer or at least some solace as I lay back on the table. "I remember what happened now," I said, stupefied. "I just can't remember his name." The minutes ticked by.

"Dillon," Maryanne said abruptly, her voice startling me.

Thrilled at her recall, I exclaimed, "Yes, that's it!" I felt as if she had found a lost treasure. "How in the world did you remember his name after all this time? You have an incredible memory!"

"I didn't remember it," she said in a correcting and seemingly irritated voice. "He just told me."

Elated, I could hardly get the words out quickly enough, "He's back? You see him again?" Her eyes were staring through the same open doorway as before, but I still couldn't see anything.

"Yes, he's back," she continued, "and he's not too happy you forgot his name."

"I am so sorry, Dillon. I will never forget your name again," I apologized to him silently.

"He has his wagon again," she reported, "and the bear." My heart pounded as I waited for each word to pass through her lips. "He's telling me he plays with Meghan a lot."

My mind raced to Meghan's incredible imagination and how she would talk to someone on her toy telephone for great lengths of time. In fact, it was the only toy that held her attention for more than five minutes. Was it possible she was talking to Dillon during that time?

Maryanne interrupted my thoughts as I heard her say, "He's telling me that one of your life's missions is to write a book." She paused. "The name of the book will be," and she paused again as though waiting to hear the name herself, "*Angel Babies.*" She paused yet again. "He's saying, 'To help heal the mommies who've lost their babies.'" Silence filled the room once again as she seemed to listen to what he was saying so that she could relate it to me. "You'll talk about the babies in the afterlife." Stunned speechless, my brain attempted to grasp what she had just said.

"I see babies going down slides into the clouds," she continued. "He's waving good-bye. He's gone."

My mind felt paralyzed by the information I'd just received. As the shock wore off, incredible emotions raced through me. I was overjoyed that Dillon had returned, and deep love filled my being as I thought of him. But as I recalled his words about writing a book, other feelings emerged—feelings of doubt and fear.

I couldn't write a book. I wasn't a writer. Didn't he know that? And I certainly couldn't write a book about baby spirits on the other side. What did I know about that? And what would people think? *They'd think I'm a nut, that's what,* I answered myself. *I am not going to write a book about the afterlife. Wrong life mission. Wrong mommy.* I let out a deep sigh. *Besides, he didn't say I must do it,* I added for emphasis.

I had remained mute through the rest of the massage. I was too busy talking to myself. I dressed quickly and joined Maryanne in the lobby, and now I had plenty to say.

"First of all," I announced, "I am not a writer. Surely, he knows that. Second," I paused, still trying to assimilate the information she had given me, "he wants me to write a book about babies in heaven?" I looked at Maryanne to see if I understood her correctly. She nodded.

"Well, what if I can't? What if I don't know how? What if this is too big for me?" I rambled. "What if I don't want to?" I asked her, wanting an answer. I stood there hoping she would give me an answer. Maryanne just looked at me without addressing any of my questions. So then I tried to make "the mission" more palatable. "What if I write about the feelings of loss with a miscarriage? Maybe I could write about that," I said, trying to find a way to accept a mission I didn't want. I felt more comfortable doing a safer assignment, where I could do my coloring inside the lines. "I don't know," I said, shaking my head from side to side. I was trying to persuade myself as much as her. "Maybe," I repeated, as my mouth contorted as though I'd just eaten something bitter. Talking about spirit babies was far too big for me to digest.

After I left, I reviewed what I had been told by Maryanne, from Dillon. I wouldn't forget anything this time or ever again. I felt a mounting surge of excitement course through me. I couldn't wait to tell Tim. I picked up my cell phone and dialed our home phone number as I said out loud, "This time he'll really listen."

As soon as I heard his voice, I told him what had happened as fast as I could get the words out. He was as astounded as I was, and more important, this time he was supportive.

The next morning, I went to my favorite bookstore to investigate books on miscarriage. I scanned the huge wall of books on pregnancy, child rearing, and parenting. Overwhelmed by the sheer volume of books, I asked a clerk if she could direct me to the miscarriage section.

A pleasant woman, Roseanne, walked over to the bookcase, reached down, and handed me what I thought was the first of many books. I was impressed by her efficiency. The book she handed me was a paperback only a quarter of an inch thick. "Here you go," she declared with the thoroughness of a job well done, and she turned to walk away.

"Wait, what about all the other books? Surely there are more books on miscarriage than this," I asked, glancing at the flimsy book in my hand and then to the many shelves of books in front of us.

"This is the only book we have on miscarriages," she said apologetically, "but we can order one if you'd like." I looked at the book she had handed me and my shoulders slumped forward. It was the same book my midwife had given me, and it dealt very little with the emotions surrounding the loss of a baby, let alone anything spiritual.

"This is the *only* book you have on miscarriages?" I asked in disbelief as my eyes scanned the hundreds of baby books. "I thought there'd be more," I added, as my voice trailed off. I mumbled to myself, "Then I guess I do have to write about it."

"You should," Roseanne declared.

"What?" I replied sheepishly, not realizing I had spoken loud enough for her to hear me.

"You should write a book about miscarriages. I had a miscarriage, and no one would talk about it. It was as though it never happened. My family told me it wasn't like it was a real baby, and it was never mentioned again."

Another customer approached her for help. "Write the book," she said, as she wandered down another aisle, out of sight. I stood immobilized as I realized no one was talking about miscarried babies.

Why is it so hard to believe that experiences like mine can happen when most religions believe in an afterlife or believe that fetuses are living souls? For reasons I don't clearly understand, validation of these experiences isn't given by many religions.

I grew up believing in a place called heaven, where good people would go when they died, but I had always thought of this place being in a distant galaxy. I had no idea then that it is really but a thin veil of consciousness that separates us from those who've passed on and prevents us from seeing through to their spirits. I came to understand much later that their souls are so close and that if we just whisper their names in our hearts, we will know they are there.

But at that moment, I needed fresh air. As I walked out into the Florida sunshine, I began questioning the odds of having a store clerk who happened to help me share her miscarriage story with me.

I walked down a few doors into a department store and was drawn to a new display of bath items. I looked at the shelf immediately in front of me and let out a gasp. My eyes froze on a plastic box containing three winged angel heads made of soap. Printed boldly on the plastic case were the words "Angel Babies."

At the time, it was rare to find anything with angels. There was no way the name Angel Babies on a soapbox was just a meaningless coincidence, and neither was my conversation with the bookstore clerk. "Okay, okay, I got it," I said out loud, not caring who might hear me, as I looked upward.

A bit shaken by the course of events, I lost interest in doing any further shopping. I walked to the check out line to buy the Angel Babies soap. I knew I'd need evidence for times when the skeptic in me emerged, as it always did. The box would offer me the proof I needed, so I'd know I hadn't imagined it.

Doubts began only a few minutes later as I drove home. Did Maryanne make up the whole thing? Maybe she was just being nice and thought she'd be helping me. Exactly who was Maryanne? Was she psychic? Could she really see and hear my baby?

What was the "you will write a book" dialogue about? Now that was way out of my comfort zone. *Well, he didn't say I had to write it,* I reassured myself. No, this was too far out on a limb for me. *Maybe Maryanne was hallucinating.*

A few more miles passed as I continued my drive home. "But I felt his presence when I spoke to him," I confidently uttered. His presence was real.

"And I heard him," I announced before adding, "twice," prior to Maryanne first seeing him. When I'd heard him I hadn't even been thinking about him. It had been totally unexpected. And I had definitely heard him, of that I was certain.

And what about the other voice asking about Meghan? I would not have made that up. I was irritated the question was even asked, and I was surprised there was someone else, or rather another spirit, intruding on our conversation.

No, there was no way I would have imagined the answer Dillon gave me. I had never even had a passing thought that I could be pregnant with twins. I certainly wouldn't have imagined that Meghan had returned to me. Sure, I thought reincarnation was a possibility, but miscarried babies returning to the same mother in another body? No, that was too much, too far beyond the depth of my understanding. *Maybe I really am going crazy.* And with that thought, I was home.

After a few months, I was feeling that I needed some kind of confirmation or clarification, and so I went for a psychic reading. A woman in my dentist's office had told me about a psychic named Kenn. She said he was really good, and I thought it might be interesting to hear what he'd say. I set up an appointment.

As I sat down at his cherry wood dining room table, I crossed my legs. "Uncross your legs," he ordered. How did he even know I'd crossed my legs, I wondered. I obediently uncrossed my legs and automatically sat up straighter.

"I'm going to ask you to shuffle the cards and place them down when and where I tell you to," Kenn continued. Obviously, he had some rules to follow. "Don't ask any questions until the end of the reading. If I haven't answered your questions, then you can ask."

Kenn began by saying, "You are going into a positive time. Books everywhere, books, books, books. You like to read."

He was right about that. My living room was more of a library. I love reading and being surrounded by books.

"You do a lot of praying," he remarked. "You haven't had the confidence, but you're getting it."

Could he mean confidence about the book? I wondered.

"Blue in all shades is important to you," he remarked.

That's true; I love the color blue but didn't comment aloud.

"There's a book you will write."

Did he say "book"? I wondered.

"You lost a child, didn't you? He was a boy. Your son is your main spirit guide."

That statement was very impressive, though I didn't tell him at that moment.

"You have a sister in spirit."

Possible, I supposed, since my mother had had several miscarriages.

"Your father-in-law, a man with a leg problem that caused him to walk with a limp, is there."

Wow, Tim's dad limped after his stroke.

"Indian forces are protecting you."

I didn't know what to make of that.

"You are very compassionate."

I guess, but aren't most people?

"You have two daughters as different as night and day. The little one is going, going, going. She looks like the drawing on this Christmas card."

I looked at the line drawing of a little girl on the Christmas card, which he picked up from the table to show me. Meghan could have been the model for it. What was unusual about it was that the little girl had short hair, like Meghan's. Most photos or drawings I'd seen of little girls that age had long hair. His card showed a little girl with light hair, cut in a short bob, just like Meghan's. Now that was good.

"Your mother and father are in spirit. They are your guides, as well as your son and Indians. Your family has become your guides. The more you talk to them, the more they will help. Your folks have to work off karma to you as a result of your childhood."

Oh, wow, I thought. Kenn wouldn't have known my parents were alcoholics whose disease led to some unhappy experiences for me as a child. It seemed that spiritually they feel a karmic debt to me.

"You think, think, and think!"

Okay, so maybe I did, but he didn't have to make it sound so negative.

"You have happiness in your home."

It certainly felt that way to me.

I had every confirmation possible, but I didn't really listen as Kenn talked about the book, my parents and Dillon being my guides, or all the other amazing information he related. I focused on how accurate he was about the drawing that looked like Meghan. Perhaps we hear only when we're truly ready to listen.

Apparently I wasn't ready to listen, and the coming holidays brought new activities to focus on. It had been eight months since I had first heard Dillon after my nap, and he was not on my mind that day. It was far too hectic to do anything except supervise eight little three- and four-year-olds as we celebrated Meghan's fourth birthday.

I picked up some dirty glasses in the living room where the children were playing and slipped away to the kitchen. Grateful for a few moments of solitude, I slowly rinsed the glasses, letting the water roll over my hands as I stood quietly mesmerized at the sink.

"Mommy?" The voice interrupted my peace. It was soft and clear and came from directly behind me.

"Yes, honey?" I replied as I turned around to see what Meghan needed. I stood alone in the kitchen. Meghan and the other children were all in the living room. Little children's voices calling "Mommy" tend to sound alike. But I know the voice had come from right behind me and had to be *his* voice.

Smiling, I replied, "Oh, Dillon! Hi, honey. Thank you for coming to Meghan's birthday party." I surprised myself with my calm response. My moment with Dillon was broken as squeals of delight came from the living room. I walked to the room filled with little girls celebrating Meghan's special day, content knowing Dillon was part of it, too.

PREGNANCY, MISCARRIAGE, AND RECOVERY

Having had several experiences of hearing from Dillon made me reflect on my brief pregnancy with him and the events that had occurred during that time.

Although my pregnancy with Dillon had been planned, a lot of confusion surrounded it from the very beginning. Perhaps the events were warning signs that the baby wouldn't be coming.

I had caught an especially bad cold and felt awful in every way, desperately wanting to take medication to relieve my symptoms—but not if I were pregnant, which I hoped I was. I decided to find my answer by taking a blood test at a nearby walk-in clinic.

When the clinic called me an hour later with the test result, I was sprawled out on my bed, my head so stuffy I couldn't breathe, fantasizing about taking my favorite cold remedy. In fact, I felt so miserable that when they told me the result was negative, I felt disappointed but not broken-hearted, which would have required far more energy than I had at the time. I couldn't wait to take a cold pill, knowing I wouldn't be harming a little one inside of me.

A week later, I became puzzled when I was four days late starting my period. I took a home pregnancy test and waited for a blue line to appear indicating I was pregnant. The line appeared, but it was barely visible. The directions read that even if a faint blue line appeared, the result was positive. I was confused. The blood test had said I wasn't pregnant. Which test was more accurate? The blood test, I assumed. Still, I couldn't get it out of my head all day; so in the afternoon, I took another home pregnancy test. It read positive.

I called the toll-free number on the box to ask about the accuracy of the test. I was assured it was 99 percent accurate, but I was afraid to get excited due to the blood test.

I called the hospital office of my midwives to find out whether I could be seen right away for another blood test. Maybe the walk-in clinic did something wrong. As soon as Kylie woke up from her nap, we made the thirty-minute drive to the hospital.

Susan, one of the midwives, listened to my story and began by giving me a urine test. It came back with a dark horizontal line indicating it was negative, but with a light vertical line making it a positive sign, giving a confusing result. "Am I pregnant or not?" I asked.

"It's positive," she said, "but let's run the blood test." Kylie and I waited in the lobby for the results while I wondered why I was having such a hard time getting a straight answer from the tests.

"The results came back negative," the nurse told me.

"Run it again," I heard Susan yell out to her from across the hall. Again we waited.

"It's positive," Susan declared confidently. "You are definitely pregnant." I burst into tears of joy. "You are four weeks and four days pregnant. The baby is due May 1," she added.

My stomach tightened when I heard the due date. Quietly, I told myself, "No, the baby will be born on May 8, because that's my dad's birthday." The next thought was unsolicited, bursting into my mind so fast that I didn't have a chance to screen it. It seemed to come from someplace other than my own mind: "The baby is my dad returning." The information startled me, and I gasped. Where had that thought come from? Suddenly, uneasiness came over me.

I reminded myself of my joy at being pregnant, dismissing my irrational thought as hormone overload and pushing the uncomfortable feeling away before stopping at the store to buy a dozen pink and blue helium balloons. I wanted to tell Tim the good news in person and see the surprise on his face. Although I knew it might give away the surprise, I tied the balloons along the driveway and added pink and blue streamers to the branches of trees as I waited impatiently for the sound of Tim driving up.

As he walked in the door, I handed him an elegant glass of clear soda, and beaming with excitement, I exclaimed, "We have something to celebrate. I'm pregnant!"

"Are you sure?" he asked hesitantly, knowing the results of the initial blood test. His response wasn't what I had expected or wanted.

"They ran the test twice just to be sure," I explained, but I felt heaviness in the air.

He too felt confused about whether I was pregnant or not. We tried to figure out why we both felt so hesitant. We decided not to tell anyone right away until we could get our feelings in check. Something held us back from getting excited.

I didn't have any sense of foreboding when I was pregnant with Kylie. Why did I feel it so strongly now? Where was this feeling coming from? Ominously, it seemed to surround my heart and lungs.

Fear emerged and suddenly molded itself into a single thought: the baby would bring me great emotional pain. Why would I have such a terrible thought, and why did I feel like crying? I knew it was an irrational fear, but I couldn't seem to shake it.

Each time I felt the fear, I'd push it away and begin to let the growing excitement of being pregnant emerge. As the days passed, the reality that I was pregnant began to sink in, and our excitement slowly grew.

Tim and I began to discuss names for the baby. I was certain it was a boy. Tim felt just as strongly that it was a girl. We focused more on boys' names because we thought finding the right boy's name might be a little harder. We wanted a strong Irish name.

We talked about the baby a lot, about how many grades apart Kylie and the baby would be in school, how many years they'd be together in elementary school, and how wonderful Kylie would be with the new baby. We talked about when we would have him or her baptized and who the godparents would be. We talked about the baby so much, imagining future times, that he or she was already a part of our family. Mostly, though, we talked about how much we already loved the baby.

We decided to add a room to the house for our new little one and contacted the bank about a loan. I began designing the baby's room in my mind and enjoyed visualizing decorative themes. I was drawn to wallpaper I'd seen with a brown bear in a sailboat. I spent long moments imagining the baby in his crib.

One afternoon, the bank called to tell us that we were turned down for the loan. I sobbed uncontrollably for what felt like a very long time, my reaction far out of proportion to the news.

"Honey, it's just a room," Tim said, trying to console me. "Where are these tears coming from?" he asked gently.

"Don't you see?" I asked belligerently. "We aren't getting the loan because we won't need the loan, because there won't be a baby!" I didn't know where the words had come from, but they seemed to convey what a deeper part of me sensed. It was obvious to me why I felt a deep sadness about not getting the loan, but Tim didn't follow my logic.

Exhausted from crying, I curled up in Tim's arms as I listened to his soothing voice assure me the baby was okay. A few minutes later, I felt a little embarrassed by my emotional outburst. Again, I chalked it up to hormones.

Continuing with happier talk, we decided to plant a tree to honor our new baby, so that as the baby grew, we'd watch the tree grow, too. We decided on a camphor tree since we knew they grow to be big, beautiful trees with strong trunks and wide branches. We planted it on the side of our backyard where it wouldn't block our view of the Gulf of Mexico. We were excited to watch it grow.

Nine weeks into my pregnancy, I had to make a business trip to Myrtle Beach, South Carolina. Tim and Kylie joined me. They played while I worked, but I loved having them close.

During the first dinner of the conference, I sat with a group of colleagues whom I knew from previous conventions and excitedly told them, "I'm pregnant!"

"Don't you know," the man seated to my side boldly scolded, "you aren't supposed to tell anyone you're pregnant until you're past the twelve-week mark? What if you had a miscarriage?" My jaw dropped to the floor, and my face become hot with embarrassment. I sat stunned by his response, feeling I'd done something terribly wrong. Everyone at the table stared at me in what felt like unending silence. Were they waiting for an answer? A foreboding feeling about the baby enveloped me once again. *What if he were right?* I wondered.

I was relieved when someone brought up the topic of the weather, breaking the dead silence at our table. I became unaware of what was being said but grateful the focus was elsewhere. Quiet and still, I went inside myself and felt growing fear and sadness.

I waited for what seemed an appropriate length of time before excusing myself from the table. Once back in my room, Tim and I went outside on the private balcony while Kylie slept peacefully. As I told Tim what had happened at the dinner table, my soft crying soon escalated to huge sobs. "What if he's right?" I asked Tim. Once again, Tim held me as he whispered positive reassuring comments about the baby being okay. I had never miscarried before, and my pregnancy with Kylie was mostly uneventful. Finally, I stopped crying. My emotions in control, I asked, "Gee, why am I so emotional?" Tim didn't have an answer, and so I surmised that my hormones were acting up yet again.

The next morning, I spotted. Panic-stricken, I called my midwife, who calmly explained, "Sometimes spotting happens when the baby is implanting on the uterine wall. It's probably nothing, but just to be sure, let's do a sonogram when you return."

For the next two days, I sat in my booth, passing out brochures, pretending everything was all right. The baby was in my thoughts constantly. I couldn't wait to get home and put my mind at ease.

The sonogram was done at the hospital where my midwives had their office. Tim and I were both anxious, not sure of what awaited us. As I lay down on the examination table, Tim lovingly caressed my hand. I looked into his green eyes to see whether they were as calm as his hands, but they were full of concern. Neither of us spoke as we watched the monitor, hoping to hear the baby's heartbeat. "Please, God, let the baby be okay," I repeated to myself, hoping my plea would make it so. The hospital room seemed deathly quiet and smelled of antiseptic.

When the technician found the baby's heartbeat, it was so loud it startled us. Tim and I both commented on how strong and sure of itself the little heart sounded. Tears streamed down my cheeks as I breathed a sigh of relief. Tim leaned down to kiss me, and I realized he was close to tears. In that moment, the baby became real. More important, the baby was alive, its little heart beating boldly and confidently. How could anything be wrong with a heartbeat that strong, we reasoned.

"Does the baby look okay?" I asked the technician, even though I knew she wasn't allowed to tell us anything.

"The radiologist needs to review the results of the sonogram first, and then he'll discuss them with your midwife," she explained professionally. She looked at our reddened eyes before adding, "But everything looks good," attempting to ease the strain. "Come back in an hour and your midwife will have the results."

Excited and relieved, we left the hospital. It felt good to breathe deeply again. We laughed as we talked about how wonderful it was hearing the thumping beat of a little heart.

Tim's office was only a few blocks away, and since the crisis seemed over, he felt comfortable attending to a few things there while I chose to go to a nearby park. I wanted to thank God for the baby being okay.

As I sat on the wooden bench, I felt a slight breeze and marveled at the beauty of the day. I replayed the baby's heartbeat over again in my mind as I expressed my gratitude to a power greater than myself. Feeling calm and relaxed, my eyes wandered up the trunk of a large oak tree and through the branches, to the top of the tree. My eyes stopped as I reached the crystal blue sky. Mesmerized, I sat breathing quietly as my mind became devoid of thoughts. I stared into the blue nothingness of the sky until my eyes tired. As I let them relax, my gaze dropped down to the scene directly in front of me.

Suddenly, a dark gray cloud mass appeared fifteen feet in front of me.

Separate and to the right was a brilliant white cloud mass. Somehow, in a way I can't explain, I instantly knew that the dark cloud represented my father's disease of alcoholism and that the white cloud represented my dad's true self. I knew with untold certainty my dad deeply loved me. I could feel his love envelope me. An understanding came over me that it was the disease that had caused me pain, not my dad. The two were separate. In what seemed like a timeless moment, I completely understood the difference between my dad and his illness. With this understanding, I felt healed.

And with that, the vision was gone. As I became aware of my surroundings again, I quickly looked around to see whether anyone else was in the park might have seen the clouds, but the park was empty.

"What just happened?" I asked myself. I felt wonderful, jubilant. My shoulders felt lighter. Words can't adequately describe the power of this vision, the love I felt from my dad, and the healing I had experienced. It was powerful and poignant beyond imagination. Years of therapy couldn't give me what I got in that one brief moment, and I couldn't wait to tell Tim what I'd just witnessed.

Feeling confident, Tim and I returned to the hospital and smiled broadly when we saw our midwife, Kathleen.

"The baby looks great," she reported with a wide smile, knowing it was the news we wanted to hear. Tim and I looked at each other with relief as all the remaining tension in our bodies melted away. We both sighed deeply, thinking the worst was over. "The only thing is," Kathleen continued with a confused look on her face, "the baby isn't as far along as we thought. The baby is five weeks, five days along, not nine and a half as you thought.

My body tensed. "Is there any way a baby can catch up in growth?" I questioned her, hoping for a positive response.

"No," she answered emphatically. My body slumped in the chair as I tried to understand.

Seeing the look of concern on my face she asked, "Could your dates be wrong?"

"Kathleen, I have never wanted to be wrong about something more than this, but I know exactly when I got pregnant. I have the home pregnancy test to prove it," I said, sounding defeated. "And you did a blood test!" I added as more proof. Quickly, my mind screamed to God for me to be wrong.

"What are you sensing?" Kathleen asked. "The mother often seems to know if the baby will be okay," she added softly.

I sensed everything would not be okay. Stunned, I looked blankly at Tim as a deep heaviness surrounded me. My chin began to quiver as my eyes filled with familiar hot tears. Sadly, I knew the outcome. My eyes returned to look at Kathleen. "Tell me what to expect with a miscarriage," I asked quietly as a low buzzing filled my head.

Kathleen took a deep breath. "There will be cramping ..." I saw her lips moving, but I no longer heard what she was saying. The buzzing in my head drowned out her words as my face became hotter and hotter. Not caring what she said, my eyes wandered to a blank place on the wall, and I felt momentarily suspended in time and space before turning again to look at Kathleen. It was as though I were watching a silent movie.

The buzzing suddenly stopped, and I heard her voice again. "Are there any questions?" Kathleen asked.

I looked at Tim, unable to comprehend what was about to happen. As we saw the pain in each other's eyes, we wept. The tears seemed to come from the very core of our souls. Kathleen quietly left the room to give us some privacy. Eventually, we collected ourselves enough to walk out to the car and drive home.

Desperately trying to find hope, I prayed fervently that I was wrong about my dates. I thought that the vision in the park had meant everything would be okay. I had let go of my fear concerning my dad and the baby. So why wasn't the baby okay? Wasn't that the purpose of the vision? Or was it the baby's gift to me before leaving? It was a wonderful gift, one I would be eternally grateful for, but it was overshadowed by fear of losing the baby.

Tim became upset with my feeling so certain I would miscarry. "We heard the baby's heartbeat," he reasoned like a lawyer, "so you should have a positive attitude. Fight for the baby."

I tried to have a positive attitude, but it felt as though I were pulling my heart behind me with a rope tied to a five-hundred-pound weight. Why was my heart not accepting what my mind said?

I prayed I was wrong about my dates. I prayed my baby would be okay. I prayed the five-hundred-pound weight would disappear and my heart would hop off the floor and back into my body. Exhausted, I prayed to lose the baby now, not later, if something were wrong. If I carried the baby longer, I might love it even more, and then it would hurt more to lose it. I was already experiencing more pain than I felt I could bear. I prayed for peace and let go of my fears as I drifted off to sleep.

When I awoke the next morning, I felt oddly at peace. The sadness had lifted. Maybe everything was going to be all right after all. I let go of any negative thoughts. This wonderful, serene feeling lasted all day, and I embraced it.

As I got undressed to take a shower that evening, the shock of seeing blood threw me against the wall. Hysterical, I called Tim's office. "Honey, it's begun," I whispered through sobs. "We're losing the baby. I'm so sorry." Suddenly, I felt solely responsible for the loss of the baby.

Tim rushed home, and we held each other through the night as waves of loss, crushed dreams, and tears came and went like the rhythm of the ocean. Tim cancelled his appointments for the next day to be with me. Our child was dying, and we wanted to be together as we went through the miscarriage.

The next morning, I awoke to the thought that this was the day we would lose our baby. Grief clutched my throat, and I began sobbing convulsively. Tim held me tenderly as we both wept uncontrollably over the loss of our baby.

Suddenly, we heard Kylie's voice call out to us to tell us she was awake. We quickly shifted our thoughts to her and the day ahead, realizing that in a matter of hours, six one- and two-year-old children would be arriving for Kylie's second birthday party. Tim and I quickly decided we didn't want to cancel the party. We wanted to celebrate Kylie's life. As the morning progressed, however, it seemed I was hemorrhaging.

In the afternoon, we gathered the children at the party to sit at the table for birthday cake, and I ran to the bathroom yet again, trying to keep my composure as I saw that I was losing my baby. When I heard the children begin to sing "Happy Birthday" to Kylie, I ran to the kitchen to see Kylie's pure delight at the sight of her birthday cake. Tim looked up, and our eyes locked, mine now brimming with tears. As Kylie blew out the flames of the two candles on her cake, I thought of the flame of our new baby's life being extinguished at the same time. Unable to hold back tears, they spilled onto my cheeks and rolled quickly down my face. I muffled a sob as I leaned on a friend's shoulder.

Hours later, when the party was over, I realized I was beginning to feel very weak. "We'd better call the doctor," I said to Tim as I sat down. "Something isn't right."

We were told to go to the hospital, and we asked a trusted neighbor to watch Kylie for us. I couldn't put on a brave front any longer and didn't want to stifle my tears. I didn't think I was strong enough.

During our thirty-minute drive to the hospital, I began rocking back and forth, trying to comfort my shaking body. Filled with fear, I began chanting the beginning of the Serenity Prayer: "God, grant me the serenity to accept the things I cannot change." Over and over, I repeated the words as a mantra.

The hospital staff was expecting us and ushered us into a private room. "You look white," Tim remarked with concern. He held my hand and gently stroked my hair as we waited for the doctor to arrive. It was obvious I was hemorrhaging now, and it was worrisome. "I think I might faint," I said softly to Tim. I had never fainted before, but I felt light-headed and very weak.

I needed a D&C, a medical procedure to clear out my womb, and was given some drugs to sleep through it. The next thing I knew, I was in another room with drapes surrounding the bed for privacy. Tim was sitting next to me, stroking my hair as I opened my eyes.

"How do you feel?" he asked softly.

"Empty," I responded slowly. Oddly, I hadn't experienced any cramping. The only pain I felt was that of my heart breaking.

Our ride home was quiet, with Tim and I lost in our own thoughts. We picked up Kylie from the neighbor's, and I held her closely, appreciating on a deeper level what a wonderful gift she was.

In the middle of the night, Kylie woke up crying. I went to her room and picked her up to comfort her. "It's okay, sweetheart. Mommy's here."

"Baby's gone. Where's baby?" she asked, sounding distressed as she looked down at the floor and then frantically around the room as though trying to find something. I thought she was referring to her stuffed animal. Baby was a white bunny she had fallen in love with from the minute she saw it in her Easter basket when she was six months old. Baby was her "lovey," who was always nearby, especially while sleeping and when she needed comfort.

"No, honey, you didn't lose Baby. You're holding Baby. See?" I said, as I pulled her hand up to show her she was holding her rabbit. She kept looking at the floor and rambling, "Baby's gone. Where's baby?" I finally calmed her down and put her back to bed, assuming she was confused during her half-asleep state.

The next night, she woke up crying again. I picked her up as she looked frantically at the floor as though she'd dropped Baby and couldn't find it. I reassured her that she was holding Baby and put her back to bed when her tears subsided.

The next morning, I sat up in bed and realized why Kylie was crying and confused. She wasn't talking about her Baby, she was talking about our baby. She had probably heard Tim or me say we had lost the baby. She thought the baby was misplaced and that if we looked for it somewhere on the floor, we'd find it. After all, that was where she'd always find her baby when it was lost. Although she was only two years old, on some level she understood the loss of the baby. Perhaps she understood far more than we realized.

The following weekend, I had to attend a training seminar for my job. We were given a worksheet to fill out at the beginning of the class.

I knew it was important, but I couldn't concentrate on something so seemingly mundane. I wrote, "Just had a miscarriage," over the top of the page. In other words, I am incapable of doing this right now. As the instructor read my paper, he looked at me briefly and then went on to the others. When he asked questions, my colleagues were giving answers with such enthusiasm that I just wanted to stand up and scream, "Don't you understand? I just lost my baby!" My boss gave me an "aren't you going to get involved?" look, and so I tried to pretend I was interested in what we were doing. So I faked it. And as the weekend progressed, I found myself laughing. It felt amazingly good to laugh again. Slowly, tentatively, I began to heal.

Our vacation time, planned months earlier, took place three weeks after the miscarriage. The timing couldn't have been more perfect. We were going to vacation at our cabin in the mountains, but one morning, as Tim was walking out the door for work, he looked back at me and paused. With a twinkle in his eye and a mischievous grin, he said, "I'm feeling a little Carib-be-an," emphasizing the syllables in a rhythmic way while his shoulders and hips swayed with the sounds. My eyebrows rose as I realized what he was suggesting. "Are you feeling a little Caribbean?" he asked me, still moving his body in a semi-dance.

"Why, I think I am," I replied and smiled.

Excited about the possible change in location, we both began singing our favorite clipped and bouncy Jamaican tune as I walked Tim to his car and kissed him good-bye.

"If you have time today, see what you can put together," he called out the car window as he backed out of the driveway.

I searched the Sunday paper to see whether any packages or specials were offered to any island in the Caribbean. I found the word "Jamaica" printed in bold type. A home in Ocho Rios was advertised for a week's rental. The house sounded too good to be true. It had three bedrooms, a pool, a full-time staff to prepare all meals, and a driver to pick us up at the airport. The rental fee was so low I was sure it was an error. I dialed the local phone number listed to clarify the price.

A pleasant-sounding woman answered the phone and said she was the owner. When I asked about the rental fee, she assured me the price listed was correct. Affordable! My excitement began to grow. When I was told the home was available during the time period we needed, I booked it on the spot.

As I hung up the phone, I sat in awe at how perfect the house sounded and how easily our Jamaican holiday just seemed to fall into place. I knew Tim would be thrilled. We loved Ocho Rios, and with a two-year-old, staying in a house would be so much easier than in a hotel room.

The house was charming. A man and a woman were waiting outside for us as we arrived. They introduced themselves as they took our luggage to the house.

"I'm Clover, your housekeeper. I'll be making your meals for you," she said in her beautiful Jamaican accent, accompanied by a bright, wide smile.

"I'm Clarence. I take care of the yard and the house," he said, smiling. Clover showed us the house before quietly disappearing.

"This is incredible!" Tim and I said in unison as we eagerly unpacked.

Clover made every meal for us, including Kylie's. It felt extravagant beyond our imagination. I felt so nurtured and taken care of, as though I were being nursed back to health.

At night, Kylie would fall asleep by seven o'clock, allowing Tim and me to eat dinner alone. Dinner was especially lovely because Clover would serve each course separately. She gave us a little bell to ring when we were done with each course, to let her know we were ready for the next one. At the beginning of the week, we felt quite shy and embarrassed to use the bell, but by the end of the week, we were ringing it with confidence. We had all our meals outside on the porch overlooking the pool, with the ocean in the distant background. It was beautiful, relaxing, and healing.

One day melted into another as Clover mothered me with her meals, and we relaxed by the pool, allowing the rhythm of our bodies to dictate when we ate and slept.

Toward the end of the week, Tim and I decided to go rafting down the Martha Brae River and left Kylie with Clover. We drifted smoothly down the same river I'd seen in an old home movie showing my parents doing the same.

"It's so strange to think my parents rafted down this river thirty or so years ago," I said to Tim before pausing a bit. "I think they were happy then." As I watched the beautiful lush scenery of the Jamaican countryside unfold around each bend of the river, I found myself lost in thought about my parents.

"Tim, do you think my parents were instrumental in our coming to Jamaica?"

"It wouldn't surprise me at all," Tim responded after thinking about it for a minute.

"It just feels like we were pulled to come here. It all fell into place so easily. Don't you find that strange?" I questioned.

"I guess we were meant to come here," Tim answered tenderly.

Back in Florida, my midwives suggested I let three months pass before trying to get pregnant again, and so we waited, allowing my body and our hearts to heal.

Six months later, on April 26, just prior to my due date with Dillon, I took a home pregnancy test and was ecstatic to discover I was pregnant again. It would be the same date four years later that I would hear Dillon for the first time.

Although we were thrilled about the new baby, we didn't tell anyone. We were hesitant, just in case *it* happened again. Perhaps if we didn't tell anyone, somehow the baby or we would be protected. The baby's due date was my birthday, and if I were to believe in omens, that certainly seemed positive.

A few days later, a friend called to tell me that Don, an astrologer I'd seen in the past, happened to be in town for the week and asked whether I wanted an appointment to see him. Since I had spotted that morning, I'd become somewhat fearful, realizing I wasn't immune to life's tragedies. Maybe Don could find out whether the baby would be okay. I wanted to know how the story would end, in order to prepare myself.

Don listened patiently as I told him of my concern for the baby before he turned on the tape recorder. "It's like the baby is making alterations so that he or she won't be just like you since the due date is your birthday," he began with his distinctive voice, "but the baby will be fine. If it is a girl, she will be big."

I felt as though a weight had been lifted from my shoulders after talking to Don. I hoped he was correct. Gratefully, my focus was on my new pregnancy. Dillon's due date of May 1 came and went without another wave of grief.

As each day passed, I felt more confident I would carry the baby to term, and the excitement of a new little one grew, as did our love for him or her. Finally, unable to keep our secret any longer, we beamed as we told family and friends. Gleefully, I added with emphasis, "and the baby's due on *my* birthday!" The emphasis implied nothing bad would happen to this baby.

Although I began to feel confident again, I was still hesitant to plant a tree for the new baby. "Let's plant a tree after the baby arrives," I told Tim as we stood on the porch. The tree we had planted eight months earlier for Dillon hadn't grown at all. In fact, it had lost all of its leaves and looked dead. Some days, looking at the dead tree both saddened and angered me.

"Tim, would you *please* cut down that blasted tree. The baby didn't live, and neither will the tree!" I exploded one afternoon.

"Okay, honey, I will," Tim replied in a reassuring voice. But he never did cut it down.

The months passed, and my pregnancy went smoothly, as Don had predicted. Then on an especially glorious morning in December, one day before my birthday, I gave birth to our daughter, Meghan.

As they placed her in my arms, I looked deeply into her eyes and took what felt like my first full breath in nine months. The fear of losing her was gone, and I exhaled fully, knowing she was at long last truly safe and, most important, alive.

As I held her close to my breast, our eyes locked, and as they did, I felt the doors of my heart, which had been somewhat guarded during my pregnancy, fly wildly open, and my heart filled with love for her. I didn't need to count her fingers or toes to see that she was okay. All I had to do was look into her deep blue eyes and know she was perfect. She had arrived. "I'm so glad you came," I whispered to her.

The next day, Tim, Kylie, Meghan, and I celebrated my birthday in the hospital. I loved having Meghan due on my birthday, but I was happy she'd arrived a day early, both to help me celebrate and so that she'd have her own special day. She was the best birthday gift I could have received.

Nurses kept poking their heads in my room throughout the day, never fully coming into the room. When it happened the fifth time, I asked, "Why do you keep peeking in and then leaving?"

"We want to see who gave birth to such a large baby," she answered, smiling. Meghan was ten pounds and eleven and a half ounces, and looked three months old. She was the second biggest baby my midwife had ever delivered. Meghan surprised all of us with her size, except perhaps Don, who had predicted that if I had a girl, she would be big.

The following spring, we planted a tree for Meghan. We chose a solid oak tree and planted it near the kitchen window, where I could watch it grow. I was certain an oak tree would grow.

Meghan was a ball of energy. Did she have an "Off" switch, I wondered? My saving grace was that she took long naps in the afternoon, and when possible, so would I. When I wasn't exhausted, I'd watch her in amazement.

Dillon's camphor tree didn't grow. It remained leafless, with thin, brittle little limbs. I was getting used to seeing its stunted growth and lifeless form. I no longer asked Tim to cut it down. It was our dead tree, a reminder of what we had lost.

LIVING SOULS

Three and a half years had passed since we lost Dillon. Meghan was now two years old and incredibly demonstrative in showing her love to us. Her kisses and hugs were numerous throughout the days, and we felt blessed to have her in our lives.

One day as I walked out on our back porch to admire a sunset, I glanced over to the now familiar dead tree. I thought I saw something green. Curious and unable to believe my eyes, I walked down the stairs and out to the yard for a closer look. I slowly reached over to touch a branch of the tree to be sure it was real. I couldn't believe it. Beautiful, new, bright green leaves were unfolding on every branch.

"How can this be? It's been dead for years," I asked in a whisper. I touched the leaves gently. "It's alive," I said aloud, totally puzzled. A wave of excitement and incredible joy came from somewhere deep inside of me and blasted out like fireworks. "It's *alive!*" I yelled out to Tim as I ran back to the house. "It's alive, Tim. The tree, it's alive!"

"What are you talking about?" he asked.

Breathless from running, I took his hands in mine and spoke slowly as you would to a young child. "The tree is alive. There are new green leaves. The tree is *alive!*"

I hoped he was grasping what I had just told him as I waited for his reaction. Tim looked at me blankly.

"Don't you see? The tree's alive, and so is the *baby* in the afterlife". I tried to get him to see the importance. It seemed so obvious, so clear to me.

Holding his hand, I coaxed him to follow me down the stairs and out to the yard to see the tree. "Look," I said, pointing to the new leaves. "It's a sign. The baby wants us to know he's okay." I had no idea why I said those words or where they had come from, but nothing inside me doubted what I had said.

"Incredible," Tim mumbled as he stared at the now healthy-looking tree.

I knew he was more perplexed about how a nearly four-year-old dead tree could miraculously come back to life than he was about the meaning of its new life, but I didn't care. As I nestled next to Tim, I spoke silently to the baby. "I know it's you, and I understand. Thank you so much."

One year later, I would hear Dillon for the first time.

More than two years after Dillon's tree first bloomed and more than a year after receiving his book message, I was still filled with resistance to the idea of writing *Angel Babies*. I needed more answers. I went for another massage with Maryanne, but I was looking for the truth more than a massage.

"Look," I started with a serious tone to my voice, "I need to ask you something, and I want you to be totally honest with me." I looked intently at her before informing her sternly, "I need to know the truth."

She looked at me quizzically. "Okay," she replied slowly.

"When you saw Dillon, did you make up your vision to make me feel better?" I didn't wait for her to answer before adding, "It's okay if you did—I just need to know."

"No, I didn't make it up," Maryanne replied earnestly.

"Well, I don't remember you saying you were psychic," I replied with disbelief in my tone. "Are you psychic?" I asked. I was going to get to the bottom of this mystery once and for all.

"I don't usually see people," she answered calmly. "Except for my guide, your son is the first spirit I've ever seen so clearly.

"Then why did you act so casual about it? Why weren't you flipping out?" I asked.

"I was flipping out," she assured me. "I had never seen anyone like that before."

I still wasn't sure. "You didn't make it up? Just tell me now before I go shimmying out on a limb, writing a book about angel babies." I sputtered out those last two words.

"I didn't make it up," Maryanne replied calmly and confidently. "I saw and heard your son."

I was surprised she wasn't more defensive considering my line of questioning. "Doesn't he realize I am not a writer, and I don't know what he wants me to write about? I don't know how to do it," I asked, flustered.

"Listen to the angel tape I sent you, and you'll be able to write," Maryanne assured me.

I had forgotten about the tape, but when she reminded me, I remembered her note, which read: "They said to send this to you to help you with your writing." I guess she thought I knew exactly who "they" were, but I could have used more clarity. I never did find out who "they" were.

As I climbed on the massage table and relaxed, I asked Maryanne, "Could you possibly be open to seeing Dillon again?" First I interrogate her, and then I ask her for a favor.

"I'll try," Maryanne responded with a smile. *She's a very kind person,* I thought, silently questioning whether I'd be that accommodating if someone had just grilled me with the kind of doubting questions I had posed.

She began massaging my leg, and a few minutes passed before she said, "I don't see anything, and I don't think I will today." My heart sank.

"Wait, I'm hearing, 'Meggie, Meggie, Meggie.'" My body came to full attention. I was certain I had referred to my daughter only as Meghan. Meggie was her nickname, used only within the family.

"He's behind a dark gray veil, sitting in a chair," she related as I held my breath, waiting for her next words. "He said he can't come because of Tootie." She paused before adding with emphasis, "And he's not too happy about it!" *Who is Tootie?* I wondered. I never did find out.

"Maybe he can't come until you get started on the book," she said.

Oh brother, there he goes again about the book, I said silently within the confines of my mind. Couldn't it be something easier?

"It should be light and about heaven specifically," Maryanne added.

How in the world do you make the loss of a baby *light?* How do you make light of a mother or a father's grief? What did I know about heaven? I took a deep breath and felt defeated.

Another year passed before I received a promotional brochure in the mail that immediately caught my attention. It was about a daylong workshop, "The Soul's Journey," being given in a town only a few hours' drive away. The featured speakers included Neale Donald Walsch, author of *Conversations with God*; Carol Bowman, author of *Children's Past Lives*; and a psychic medium, John Edward.

I had read *Conversations with God* and *Children's Past Lives*, and both books had a great impact on me. I was particularly excited about hearing Carol Bowman's talk, since after reading her book, I began thinking about becoming a hypnotist myself. I liked the fact that she was a mother telling her story. Her experiences with her children catapulted her into researching children's previous lives and writing about them. Her book deeply resonated within me. It would be years before I'd realize I was moved by her work because I, too, would be a mother telling my story. At the time, however, I had occasionally thought about the book I was told to write but had done nothing substantive.

Although the chief reason I wanted to attend had been to meet Carol Bowman to ask her about doing past-life work with children, as I looked at the brochure more closely, I became very interested in the psychic medium, John Edward. It was prior to the publication of his best-seller, *One Last Time*, and his television show, *Crossing Over with John Edward*. Although he was being touted as world-renowned, he was unknown to me. Just the fact that he was a real medium was good enough for me. I wanted to know about writing the book. Had Maryanne been accurate in all she'd told me?

I immediately phoned and spoke with a registrar to attend the conference. "Is it at all possible to get a private reading with John?" I asked.

"No, he will only be reading the group because he never knows who will come through," the woman answered apologetically.

"I lost a baby," I blurted out, "and I need to talk to someone who is qualified to confirm some information I've received." I hoped she'd hear the desperation in my voice.

"Let me give you the name of another psychic who will be doing readings at the conference," she said kindly before adding, "She's good. Her name is Gail Rhoads." I wrote Gail's name on the edge of the brochure, but I was disappointed it wouldn't be John.

"Thank you," I responded graciously, hoping she would hear the gratitude in my voice.

"Maybe if I point you out to John, he can help you," she added. "Introduce yourself to me in the morning before we get started."

"Thank you. Thank you so much," I said eagerly.

The conference was less than a month away. The possibility of hearing from Dillon through John was often on my mind. At least once each day, I'd mentally ask Dillon to make himself known to John, and I was certain he would.

The conference arrived, and during the morning break, I met a woman named Brenda and seemed to connect with her as we talked. The topic of psychics came up, and she told me a very good one had come to the conference.

"Really? Who?" I asked curiously.

"Gail Rhoads," Brenda responded.

"Her name sounds familiar," I said as I pulled out my brochure with a name scribbled in the corner. "Wow, someone else gave me her name, too, but I'm hoping to hear from Dillon through John."

"You might want to set up an appointment with Gail—just in case John doesn't read you," she advised.

Although I was certain Dillon would be coming through John, I decided to err on the side of caution and set up an appointment with Gail as back up.

Brenda joined me in the front row seats as we continued our conversation. I began to get nervous as we waited for John Edward to begin his talk. When he walked on stage, I recognized him from his promotional photo. He reminded me of my brother-in-law. Not only did he feel familiar, but he also had a wonderful sense of humor. I was confident I'd receive a message from him about Dillon and that I'd believe him.

"Let's begin," John said as he rubbed the palms of his hands together and took a deep breath. I sat frozen in anticipation of what would happen next. Three long weeks had passed waiting for this moment.

He walked over and stood in front of me, only a few feet away. "Someone in this area has lost a baby," he began as he held out his hand to indicate it was in the area where I was sitting. My heart beat furiously as my sweaty hand shot up.

He looked directly at me and said, "No, it's not for you."

My heart stopped beating for a moment, and my mind went numb as John addressed a man, two seats over from me. He had lost two children who had died soon after their births. As John spoke of the children, I watched the large man break down and sob. I felt deeply touched by the messages from the children to their father and was overwhelmed at what I was witnessing.

Another child came through to a foster mother. It was so moving to know the children were able to contact us and that they were still watching what was going on in the lives of those they had left behind. Riveted to my chair, I waited patiently for Dillon to come forward.

Suddenly, it was over. As John walked off the stage, I realized Dillon wouldn't be coming. Weeks of anticipation had been shattered, and tears welled in my eyes. I desperately attempted to keep huge sobs from emerging as my throat tightened. Not only was I devastated Dillon hadn't come, but I felt ashamed that I wasn't more appreciative of the process and happy for those who obviously needed to receive messages. John had said those who receive the messages are the ones who are supposed to receive them. I tried convincing myself that I shouldn't be sad, but I couldn't stop my deep feeling of disappointment.

Brenda looked at me and saw my unmasked pain. "Remember," she said, smiling, "you have an appointment with Gail Rhoads."

"Oh, yeah," I mumbled, thinking how fruitless that meeting would be. If Dillon hadn't come through John, why would he come through Gail?

I shuffled to her booth in the back of the room, introduced myself, and plopped down on the chair. I no longer had any expectations. In fact, I thought meeting with Gail was futile and a waste of money.

Gail had long, pale blonde hair that nearly touched her waist. Fascinated, I wondered whether she were once a hippie. As I eyed her up and down, I sighed deeply and wondered whether I'd believe anything she would tell me. But I needed Maryanne's messages from Dillon validated.

I never doubted I had heard Dillon speak. I had felt his presence. What I was resisting wholeheartedly was Maryanne's reporting of the mission: writing the book. I hadn't heard it directly from him, only through her. I still didn't know what he wanted me to say about babies in the afterlife.

Gail scooted her chair closer to mine, and our knees touched. My body arched back a little as my eyes tried to adjust to her being so close. She invaded my space, and I felt a little uncomfortable.

She began swaying slightly from right to left, and as she did, the long hair framing her face fell forward and swayed with her. *Why couldn't I get someone more normal-looking?* I wondered. My mind relaxed as I stared at her, hypnotized by her slowly swaying hair.

"You have a healing glow around you," she began. "Are you thinking of starting your own business?" she asked. Not waiting for an answer, she continued, "Do it. You are a healer."

Okay, so becoming a hypnotist would involve having my own practice, but who hasn't thought of having a business? Too vague, I reasoned. I answered Gail with a short "hmm," slightly bored.

"Your grandfather is here, mother's side," she reported.

I had no memory of my grandfather since he had died shortly after I was born, but my uncle had told me that when my grandfather got close to people, he would pinch them. That practice didn't endear him to me, and so when Gail said he was present, my internal response was, "Oh great, the *pincher* is here." I kept my poker face.

"No, I think it's your great-grandfather," she continued. I liked the sound of great-grandfather better. Besides, I hadn't heard anything negative about him. Still, I gave her no indication that his presence made a difference to me.

"He's saying, 'Write the book! You've been talking about it for years,'" she exclaimed with an enthusiastic smile.

My eyes widened. "Will he help me?" I blurted out.

"He says he'll help you." She paused as before she continued, "but you don't need it."

"Did you know you lost a son?" she asked as she looked past my right shoulder.

With that, my body flew back in the chair, and my jaw fell open as tears welled in my eyes.

"His eyes are like yours. There's a photo of you when you were pregnant with him. Your head is at an angle. His eyes look like yours in that photo. He has an unusual name," and she paused again as though trying to hear it. "It begins with a D." My heart was racing. "He's holding a brown, furry dog from your childhood," she continued. I knew the dog she was talking about, and I was thrilled to hear he was with Dillon.

"There's a man with black wavy hair who says he's your father," she related as her eyes now looked to my left. My dad did have black wavy hair, at least before it grayed, but I had no memory of him with it black. Gail paused again, and then said, "He doesn't know what to make of me." She was slyly grinning as she looked at me. I knew with certainty she was talking to my dad because I didn't know what to make of her and her swaying hair. He would have felt the same.

"He's saying, 'Go back to school.'" Again, I knew without question my dad was present because he was a strong proponent of education. When I completed my bachelor's degree, he encouraged me to get my master's degree. It was definitely something my dad would say to me.

If my great-grandfather, my father, Dillon, and even my dog had shown up, there was someone else I wanted to hear from. I thought I might taint the reading by asking, but I no longer cared. "Is my mother here?" I asked.

Gail's eyes seemed to be scanning the room behind me before she saw her. "Yes, she's here," she acknowledged, "but she's not with your dad." She was looking to my right, on the other side of Dillon. My parents divorced long before their deaths, and so it made sense to me that they'd not be together. "They came separately," Gail continued, "but for the same reason. They came to see you."

"She doesn't know what to make of me either," Gail said, laughing. *Bingo! That's my mom.* Gail continued with a very personal, emotionally charged message from my mother, apologizing to me for events that had happened in my childhood. I felt a little annoyed that my mom was wasting precious time apologizing when there was so much more we could talk about during this brief time. I had forgiven her, and I was sure she knew that. "It's okay, Mom," I told her in my mind. "Thank you for your apology, but I've already forgiven you. I'm okay, Mom, I've healed!" I wanted to hear about other things. Did she like Tim? Did she know I was a mother of two little girls? There were so many things I wanted her to comment on, but obviously an apology was very important to her. She never had the chance to do so in life and wasn't going to miss this opportunity.

"In three weeks, something will happen to change your beliefs," Gail said. I assumed she meant my religious beliefs, but since they had changed so drastically in recent years, I couldn't imagine what more could change. I figured she was wrong about this prediction and immediately dismissed it as inaccurate, even though she was right about everything else.

The reading ended, and I thanked Gail profusely. She wasn't the messenger I wanted or expected, but she told me everything I needed to know—and more. Maryanne was right after all.

I left Gail's booth. Too stunned to walk very far, I found a nearby seat and began to write down everything she had told me. My fine motor skills seemed temporarily hampered, making the transfer from head to paper a difficult task.

Three years later, while cleaning out some of my files, I stumbled across the notes of my reading with Gail. I began reading my scribbled words, sure that I had remembered everything Gail had said during her reading, at least everything important. As I read my notes, I stopped short at the last line. "Something will happen in three weeks to change your beliefs," I read out loud. I had forgotten Gail's prediction because I didn't understand how it applied to me.

Curious, I pulled out my old planner, opened it to the month of the workshop, and counted forward three weeks. My eyes fell to a name I had circled, and I gasped as I read "Carolene Heart." She was a past-life regressionist I had met at the Soul's Journey workshop. As I looked at the appointment time circled on my calendar, memories of my experience with Carolene flooded into my consciousness. What I discovered that day had, in fact, shaken me to my core.

Carolene had graciously welcomed me into her home. I had looked forward to my appointment with her not only for the regression experience but also to ask her about my becoming a hypnotist. We spoke leisurely for several hours before the topic of my miscarriage came up. As I talked about the loss of the baby, I felt my chin quiver and my eyes well with tears. Carolene solemnly looked at me. "Would you be willing to be the voice of Dillon?"

"Excuse me?" I responded, even though I had heard her perfectly. I swallowed hard.

"Would you be willing to be the voice of Dillon?" Carolene repeated.

"Yes," I replied politely without skipping a beat, as if what she had just suggested was normal. I didn't want to give any indication I was shocked at her suggestion and hoped my eyes were still in my head as my inner mind kept screaming, "Do *what?* She wants you to do *what?*"

I excused myself under the guise of needing to use the restroom, but what I really needed was to quiet my mind. I looked at myself in the mirror, took a deep breath, and then slowly mouthed the words, "She wants me to be the voice of Dillon." I bent over and splashed some water on my face.

I quickly thought about the grief work I'd done to heal from the loss of the baby, and I felt angry and betrayed by my tears. Hadn't I healed? Exactly how many layers of pain were there? Why did we have to work on that issue? As I dried my face, I looked at myself in the mirror one last time before opening the door.

Carolene showed me to what looked like a massage table. I obediently lay down, never sharing any of my thoughts or fears with her. I knew that if I avoided looking at a feeling, it meant I probably needed to, which really irritated me in this case.

Maybe Carolene could help heal the pain once and for all. I liked her and felt safe with her. When she told me to close my eyes and take a few breaths, I did so. After hypnotizing me, she began. "Dillon, who are you?"

I didn't see or hear an answer, and so I didn't answer her. In fact, I wasn't convinced I was hypnotized.

"Dillon, who are you?" she repeated.

Again, I didn't hear an answer, so I remained mute and wondered what, if anything, would happen. Shouldn't I be relaxed more deeply?

"Harlan," she asked of my dad's spirit, "what is your relationship with Dillon?"

"We are one," was the immediate answer in my inner mind.

What? I didn't like that answer and so I didn't answer her. I was going to wait for another answer, one I liked.

"Harlan," Carolene began again with a no-nonsense tone to her voice, "what is your relationship with Dillon?"

"We are one," came instantly and clearly to me, but again I remained silent. Surely there was another answer, I mused to myself.

"Harlan," Carolene began again forcefully.

Gee, she's not going to let go of this, I thought, somewhat irritated with her tenacity. The words "we are one" repeated in my head, and surprisingly, out they came through unexpected, heaping sobs.

Carolene began questioning my dad directly. "Harlan, why did you want to come back?"

I was curious what his answer would be, but before I could finish my own thought, I began speaking words that seemed to come from a deeper place within me.

"To help her understand, to feel her love again, physically." I felt a wave of love wash over me with his words. The words had come from my mouth and with my voice, but they didn't feel like my own. It was as though I were a bystander observing and listening to the conversation between Carolene and my father.

"I know how to come back to her, and I'm excited," Harlan continued, "but then I found another way to help her understand. It is my greatest gift to her, yet doing so means I cannot return to her. I do this for her, as my love is so great. It means I won't be with her again physically." He paused. "Still, I love her enough to do this for her. It is my greatest gift to her."

Hearing his words, I wept uncontrollably, knowing with certainty they had not come from me. I was overwhelmed. I felt his excitement as he talked about finding a way to help me understand. I also felt his disappointment (or was it mine?) since he knew he would not come into physical form, and then his total ecstasy about the gift he was to give me by not coming. Most of all, I felt the incredible depth of his love for me—far beyond anything I'd imagined. It radiated through every nerve of my being and enveloped me. It felt as though he had made a decision to put my needs ahead of his own when he decided not to come. The gift he was to give me far surpassed his taking physical form.

Once emerged from hypnosis, I had to leave immediately to pick up Meghan from pre-school before it closed. The drive took nearly an hour. There was no time to process my session with Carolene.

I was physically exhausted and emotionally astounded by the

information I'd received and experienced. That night, I fell into a deep sleep.

Upon awakening, when I reflected on my session with Carolene. I thought the understanding, the gift my dad referred to, was the vision in the park. It had been so miraculous, and I felt such healing from it, but his gift, as I was to learn, was much bigger than even that event.

THINKING ABOUT THE BOOK

As much as I wanted to, I couldn't stop thinking about the book, knowing that its focus had to be much more acceptable to me. I certainly wasn't going to write about hearing my miscarried baby. That would be too incredible.

I thought about the book, and sometimes I even thought about writing the book. I attempted to write my version of it several times, never getting past the first few paragraphs, and even those were written with great struggle. My version of the book had more to do with the grief of losing a baby, which, at the time, seemed far more plausible than talking about babies in heaven.

Sometimes I even spoke about the book, but only to a few people who I thought were safe enough to discuss such a matter—people who wouldn't think I was totally crazy, or at the very least, wouldn't tell me so to my face. I always ended the conversation by telling them why writing what Dillon suggested was ludicrous. My idea was more acceptable, more reasonable, and more, well, sane.

Several years passed, and I hadn't written so much as a page. I had done nothing, or so I thought. What I had accomplished was a vast amount of reading on everything from angels to near-death experiences to past-life regressions. Each book I read made more and more sense to me. I felt comforted by the information. Insatiable, I had another book ready to read the moment I closed the cover of the current book. I felt compelled to keep reading, and I felt my soul open during this time of many spiritual awakenings. For the first time in my life, I loved feeling truly connected to a higher source.

While exploring a new bookstore that had opened nearby, I found myself in the parenting section, glancing at book titles as I slowly walked down the aisle. One book was turned to show its full cover. As I read the title, I stopped abruptly and gasped as I picked it up. It was about miscarriages. Quickly, I skimmed through the pages of stories about mothers who'd miscarried, mothers whose link was the grief they all shared. I put the book back, sighing as I realized it was the book I thought I should have written.

A feeling of relief swept over me as I silently exclaimed to myself, *Thank God I didn't have to do that!* It felt as though I'd just avoided being hit by a truck. But my relief was short-lived, being quickly replaced by a deep sense of disappointment, which took me by surprise. I thought I had missed an incredible opportunity, personally and spiritually. I hadn't pushed myself, and as a result, I'd missed a chance for growth. *Why hadn't I written the book?* I asked. An answer came immediately from a deeper part of me. I hadn't lost a chance to grow because that wasn't the book I was supposed to write. That was my version of the book, but not the one Dillon had told me to write.

Dillon wanted me to talk about life after life, about babies growing up in heaven. Perhaps I hadn't lost my chance. My heart skipped a beat at this thought. I could still write the book even though I continued to have plenty of doubt and fear. After years of reading about spiritual matters, I felt comfortable in the knowledge I'd acquired. I left the bookstore yearning to grow and challenge myself. Maybe I could go out on a limb, after all. Maybe I could write *Angel Babies*.

I decided to do some research to find other women who'd not only been through the pain and loss but also might have communicated with their lost babies. I couldn't be the only one having such experiences, I reasoned. I'd just have to find out.

But needing more confirmation of my own experiences in order to feel more confident before I got started, I consulted a number of psychics for any additional or validating information.

While visiting my dear friend Alice on Florida's east coast for a few days, she suggested I visit John Rogers, who refers to himself as a professional medium. I was able to see him right away.

John began the reading by telling me, "You are a very nice person, a good person, very sensitive, empathetic."

So who isn't? I thought. Rather a blanket, unimpressive statement.

"I'm not saying that to be nice," he continued. "I've had many hard and mean people, and I tell them so. You should always ask for protection because you can absorb a lot of energy around you including negative energy. I see many guides around you. The faith of your childhood no longer exists. You are on a new path. They are showing me that you are very busy. They don't understand how you can think of three things at once and suggest you slow down."

I laughed nervously, knowing the truth of his statement, but then again, what mother doesn't multitask?

I was delighted when John said my husband's father and grandmother were present, because I'd been very close to both of them. Yet suddenly I blurted out, "I had a miscarriage."

"Your son is standing on your left," John announced. "He's very blonde. He is saying that he is often in the room that isn't used much. It's the room that's predominantly white."

Our formal living room is mostly white and isn't used much.

"He watches the girls from there," John continued.

Situated across from our family room, the living room would be a great location to watch the girls play.

"I'm being told that his not coming was a sacrifice," John related.

I told John about my vision in the park. "Is that the sacrifice he's referring to?" I asked.

"No," he answered. "It's something else—something bigger."

The next month, a friend called to tell me about a psychic intuitive named Christine Riley who'd given her a good reading. Tim surprised me by suggesting we see her together.

Dillon was on my mind as we walked up the stairs to her front door. When we sat at the table on her porch, she turned on the tape recorder and began by telling us, "There is a major transformation going on. Has there been a death in the past?"

"No," I answered, thinking she had meant a recent death.

"It involves endings and beginnings," she continued. "The spirit views it as significant. Sometimes when we are in it, it doesn't seem as poignant."

"I have goose bumps," I remarked.

"I do, too," she answered. "Goosebumps are a confirmation," she added. "You seem to be doing very well with this major transformation. It forces change on you. If you do so without resisting, it goes well. Absolute success, victory is coming to you, but the number seven is coming up, which means to wait. All your ducks are in a row; you've done the groundwork. A little more waiting, a little more patience—a period of time has to go by, and then it will happen." She paused and then asked, "How long ago did your mother pass on?"

"Over twenty years ago," I answered.

"Oh, it can't be that," she paused. "Oh, he's a perfect mate. Isn't that nice. Very rare you know," she remarked as she looked at Tim and me.

"You should write! You are born with the energy of expression. Part of you may be fearful, but push through it. You will be extremely successful. It has to do with communication. So it's in the writing area. Positive changes for yourself and other people," she said as she flipped over another card.

"This is the most powerful card," she continued, "the diamond. I would strongly encourage you to write. There doesn't seem to be confidence in this arena. So you have to fight through the barriers. Life purpose does not always come easily. This is part of your path. This usually comes to people with your vibration in midlife. You are hard on yourself, and you are a worrier. You doubt yourself, but no one else does. There is great strength around you, strength in marriage, in the work. The only restriction you have is the worry and doubt you place on yourself."

"What about the baby we lost?" I asked, unable to wait any longer to hear about Dillon.

"It would have been a Taurus. You were given a reason, weren't you? There was something wrong with the child, a total imbalance. I almost want to say brain stem."

I had no way of knowing whether the information about the brain stem was correct, but had he been born, the baby would have been a Taurus, just as my dad was.

"It was a he, was it not?" she asked. "That was the death I was referring to, because you came here with that on your mind. You see you have your own psychic ability. What a gift was given to you!"

The reading continued with pertinent information for Tim. We left her home shaken by the accuracy of the reading and what we had been told.

Although I was never one of those people who holds the winning ticket in any drawings, to my great surprise, I won a reading with Yvonne Gangone, while attending a conference several month's later. She resided in New York and I in Florida, and so I was delighted when she told me she could do the reading by phone. Yvonne and I had never met.

When the reading began, she told me she drew the empress card and began describing me as "pregnated," which she interpreted as developing and writing the book, as well as "full of abundance, very loving, very successful, very balanced." She then pulled another card and said, "I see a light-haired boy, a child maturing, a prize, a treasure from the sea. When we pass over, we mature. This child is watching over you. He's with your father, watching over you. This was an agreement. The choice was right. He felt he could do more for you on the other side. He doesn't want you to feel bad. He speaks of his little sister. He's with her. He has a rocking horse. She would understand this."

We had a rocking horse that Meghan loved. I have a baby picture of her on it, one of my favorite photos of her.

"He's saying 'Meghan.' I see her as tall. Old soul. She sees her brother and feels him. It's a little confusing. No one else sees and feels." I was speechless, amazed by what I heard.

She then drew the inventor card. "The one who creates. Yes, you are to write. Your son is with you on this, too."

Next, she pulled the fortune card. "You will be successful at it. The challenge is to give yourself permission. Sit in mediation. He will come."

"He's saying Meghan will be okay. Special children are not seen for who they really are. She is very loving and very sensitive. She's having auditory problems because she walks in both worlds. She hears the other side, like twenty thousand people speaking at once. Very perceptive. Meghan and her stuff are to keep you grounded. The book will have to do with Meghan, too. He wants effects on the siblings. I see a lot of blue light and white light."

She pulled the illumination card next. "Hands out. Keep writing. Don't judge yourself. Write what you feel. Validation for husband—there's something about his shoe, one shoe. Tell daddy about the shoe." A day earlier, Tim had discovered a hole in the sole of one of his shoes, and we laughed about it.

I thanked Yvonne profusely before hanging up the phone and absorbing all that she had told me. The reading resonated deeply.

The next day I checked my e-mails to find Yvonne had written me after our phone session, stating:

For some reason, sometimes after a session I still receive messages, maybe because I wasn't really ready to hang up with you, but I had to pick-up my four-year-old son from school.

Your son says, with a serious look on his face, tell Kaylie or Caleigh (spelling out the names) that he did not forget about her; we just ran out of time. I don't know who she is but I'm getting a sister or something like that. He mentions a bunny for her. I don't know what it means, but he was real adamant about it. "A bunny," he says, and shows me a white one with one black spot over the right eye and says it with a smile.

He was referring to Baby, Kylie's beloved white toy bunny with black glassy eyes.

He also wants me to tell you that your parents were there for you yesterday, but they did not get a chance to speak because Dillon felt it was important for him to reach out to all of you with a shared message that he not only was but also is a part of the family and your everyday life. Acknowledging your husband's shoe and the rocking horse is his way of saying to each of you individually that he is a part of your daily lives. He wants you all to know that he is with you.

Several months after the readings, while in mediation, and quite by surprise, I saw Dillon for the first time. He was about fifteen feet away from me, with his shoulders slumped forward and his head hanging down. His posture told me he was very disappointed about something. I yearned for him to look up so I could see his face clearly.

Then I heard him slowly speak. "It's okay, Mommy," he said with a tone that indicated he was very sad. "You don't have to write the book." Startled, my eyes popped open.

Guilt enveloped me. It really bothered me that I had let him down. "Oh, Dillon," I began. I paused, hating that I seemed to have disappointed him. I then took a deep breath and told him, "Okay, okay, I'll write the book," like a mother giving into a child's plea for a toy. I didn't want to disappoint Dillon. This seemed the one thing, perhaps the only thing, I could give him.

"Okay, I'll do it, but you better help me." And so, I took a leap of faith and became serious about writing the book.

Researching Angel Babies

The weeks passed quickly. Believing I couldn't be the only one having experiences of hearing from my baby, I wanted to find others. I began by contacting the organization founded to explore the psychic readings of Edgar Cayce, the Association for Research and Enlightenment in Virginia Beach, Virginia. I knew a publication went to its members, who might be open and willing to speak of such experiences, and I wrote asking for their stories. I also placed an advertisement in *Mothering* magazine to ask for mothers' stories. They began arriving almost immediately. Their contents were powerful reinforcement for me to continue researching and begin writing. Stories came from mothers, fathers, other family members, and friends who had been contacted by lost babies.

I had set up a post office box and an e-mail address to receive the stories. Selecting Angelbabies as an e-mail address was easy. When approval for the name came back, five numbers had been added: Angelbabies10527. Irritated, I wondered how in the world I would ever remember the numbers.

Coincidentally, I'd had a conversation with a man who told me he kept seeing the same numbers throughout his life and wondered what they meant. I thought about numbers that seemed to be constant in my own life, and I became curious about the numbers assigned to Angelbabies. I didn't really expect them to have any meaning, and I knew little of numerology. Suddenly, as I looked at the numbers, I saw it: 105 was 10-5, or October 5. My jaw fell open as I gasped and nearly fell off my chair. October 5 was the date I had miscarried Dillon. "Oh my God," I exclaimed as the hair on the back of my neck stood at attention and goose bumps covered my body. That was far beyond a mere coincidence. I felt the numbers were a message from heaven. But why was twenty-seven important? February 7 had no meaning. I just couldn't put it together.

It would be years before I'd discover the real meaning of twenty-seven. While cleaning a long-neglected bookshelf, I found Dillon's baby calendar. I was curious about what I could have possibly written in the short time I was pregnant. On the first page, my eyes fell to the small, round sticker stating, "I'm pregnant." It was placed on the twenty-seventh, the day I found out I was pregnant. The hair on my arms stood on end when I finally understood. The numbers signified the dates Dillon came and left.

It didn't take long at all for me to accumulate letters from parents and other relatives and friends. Their personal stories had profound meaning. They kept coming, and I kept careful track of each and the kind of experiences they revealed. I quickly decided not to worry about my writing skills. If *they* could give me a number like that, then *they* could help me write the book.

All the while, my own experiences continued. Some validated the need for the book or kept directing me toward that goal. One night, in a dream, I found myself seated in front of a long cherry-colored conference table in what seemed to be an office boardroom. Three men, who appeared to be in their sixties, sat across the table from me. A fourth man, obviously in charge of the meeting, spoke to me as he walked back and forth behind the seated men. I was being given instructions for something that felt important.

"They will be overseeing your new job," the fourth man told me, motioning to the men who looked purposefully at me. I sensed they had a vast amount of experience, and I felt certain they could help me since I knew they had much wisdom. "This man," he said as he put his hand on the shoulder of the man in the middle, "will work the closest to you. He will be your mentor."

The man in the middle was seated directly in front of me. I looked intently at him and began to take in his features as if memorizing them. Starting at the crown of his head, I noticed his gray hair with a slight wave at the top. I lowered my eyes slowly and focused on the horizontal lines creasing his forehead before my eyes moved down to meet his. He looked directly at me. His eyes had a particularly kind look about them.

I was struck by how intensely blue they were and said to myself, *They're so blue. They are beautiful and kind eyes. Wait, they seem familiar somehow.* The scene then quickly vanished as I realized the reason his eyes were so familiar to me. I was looking at my father.

How did I not recognize him sooner? If only he'd spoken, I would have known his voice. When I suddenly woke up, I felt as though I had been crying for a long time. I felt disappointed I had missed an opportunity to reach out to my father.

What was odd was that I had no memory of crying in my dream as I usually did when I had this same feeling. As I lay in bed, I tried to assimilate my dream. The beautiful blue color of my dad's eyes was so vivid, and it was all so real. I quickly felt that it wasn't a dream at all. My dad would be overseeing my new job, writing *Angel Babies.* I smiled, knowing he was a wordsmith and any assistance he could give me would be most welcome. After becoming more alert, I realized it was April 12, my parents' wedding anniversary.

While my spiritual experiences went on, my daily activities, revolving around the needs of my family, also continued. One afternoon, as I watched Meghan work with her speech therapist through a one-way mirror, I felt a tug at my heart. Meghan had been going to auditory processing and sensory integration therapy two times a week for nine months. It was not something she looked forward to after a long day in first grade. She was working so hard trying to pronounce words with an R in them, but I could see her frustration.

Feeling she needed additional help, or maybe I needed help, I decided to pray. I asked God to send her angels and guides to assist her. Almost as an afterthought, not wanting to leave any stone unturned, I pleaded with Dillon to help his sister. "She needs help, Dillon. If there's anything you can do for her, would you?"

Suddenly, I remembered Dillon's words: "I'm right here. I'm right here!" Any thoughts I had that Meghan had actually spoken those words quickly vanished as I realized it would have been impossible. Meghan couldn't say R. She would have pronounced the words as "I'm wight heah!" It further validated my experience of hearing Dillon.

On the way home, we stopped to pick up Kylie, who was playing at Rebekah's house. Rebekah was Kylie's best friend, and her sister Moriah was Meghan's. Kylie, Rebekah, and Moriah were in the middle of making people out of popsicle sticks.

Art was Meghan's least favorite thing to do. She struggled with visual spatial issues and fine motor skills. She couldn't translate to paper what she saw in her brain, and it usually led to great frustration, disappointment, and sometimes tears. Even coloring, which most children love to do, wasn't fun for her.

I drove the car into their driveway, and Moriah put her head in the window to ask whether Meghan could join them while they finished their projects. While I thought about the possible emotional outcome, Meghan surprised me by practically flying out of the car. I should have known she would jump at any opportunity to spend time with Moriah, even if it included a dreaded art project.

When I returned to pick up the girls, all four of them came running up to the car, anxious to show me their stick people. Although Meghan was in the back of the crowd, I was pleased she wasn't crying or looking frustrated.

"Did you do one, Meghan?" I asked, hoping I sounded upbeat, but I was concerned her answer would bring tears. The girls stepped aside to allow Meghan to come forward. She was beaming with pride as she handed me a piece of paper. I looked at her smiling face and remarked, "It looks like you decided to do something different."

She shook her head up and down, looking pleased with herself. I carefully opened the folded piece of notebook-sized paper and realized she had made a drawing. Meghan almost never drew pictures, and the few times she had in preschool, she didn't want to show them to us. I tried not to look too surprised.

She had drawn five people. Although they were primitive stick people, her use of color amazed me.

"Meghan, please tell me about your beautiful picture. Who are these people?" I asked.

Excitedly she explained, "That's you, Mommy. That's me," she said as she pointed to each person in the drawing, "that's Dillon, that's Kylie, and that's Daddy."

Hearing her use Dillon's name jarred me. It was the first time she had ever referred to the baby I lost, let alone by name.

Meghan had been made aware of Dillon's name only within the last year. I had purposefully *not* mentioned his name because I was certain one day she would tell me she was talking to a little boy named Dillon on a toy phone she loved, the one toy that held her attention. She would speak on it throughout the day with great animation, telling whoever was listening about her day. If I asked her who was on, she would quickly respond, "Ah, no one," and end the conversation. If she were talking to Dillon, it was their secret and one she guarded well. Impatient after three years of waiting for her to tell me who was on the other end of the phone, I began using Dillon's name.

"Did you say *Dillon*, sweetheart?" I asked for clarification since I wasn't sure I had heard her correctly. She had never talked about Dillon before, and his name hadn't been mentioned for many months, a lifetime to a young child.

"Yes, Mommy, Dillon. See, on the back, I wrote everyone's name," she declared proudly. Sure enough, she had written them all, including Dillon's, spelled D-e-l-e-n.

My eyes welled with tears. I looked lovingly at Meghan and said, "Thank you, darling. Thank you for thinking of Dillon." Puzzled I added, "Honey, what made you think of him?"

"He just popped in my mind, Mommy," she answered in a matter-of-fact tone.

I looked back at her drawing. Dillon was in the center of the family. He had what looked like a halo on his head.

"What were you drawing on Dillon's head, sweetheart?"

"I was trying to give him red hair, but it didn't look right."

"I think it looks perfect," I responded, although I couldn't get over the fact that Meghan had drawn a picture.

"Why didn't she do a stick person?" I asked Sue, Rebekah and Moriah's mother.

"She wanted to draw a picture," Sue responded.

"She *wanted* to draw a picture?" I repeated.

"Yes, she asked for paper and crayons," Sue answered.

As I cooked dinner and got the girls ready for bed, I couldn't get the drawing out of my mind. It was the first time Meghan had ever drawn a picture with pride, and this one had Dillon in it. What had inspired her to do something she didn't usually like to do? Why now? Why today? I stood at the stove, mindlessly stirring the spaghetti sauce, when an answer came to my mind. I had talked to Dillon just hours earlier and had asked him to help her, but Meghan didn't know about my plea. Then it hit me that it was more than a drawing. It was a message from Dillon, an acknowledgement of sorts. It was his way of saying he'd heard the request and was on the job.

Meghan's family portrait has since been framed and has hung on our kitchen wall for years. She has never drawn another.

Given what I thought was a measure of success in appealing to Dillon to help Meghan, I decided to try talking to Dillon using self-hypnosis. I put myself into an altered state and visualized an elevator going down ten flights to deepen the state. As I reached the bottom floor, the doors opened and, amazingly, Dillon was standing there.

He was so excited to see me. He lunged towards me, wrapping his arms around my waist as I dropped to the floor to scoop him onto my lap and hold him. He nestled his body close to mine, wrapping his arms and legs around me. His head came just under my chin as I embraced him for the first time and exclaimed repeatedly, "I love you, Dillon." I was thrilled to see him, imagination or not, and it felt so good to feel his little body for the first time. I repeatedly kissed the top of his head. His face was close to my chest. As I looked down at him, I noticed his lips. They seemed narrower than his sisters' were. That surprised me, and I wondered from whom he had inherited them before realizing they were like mine.

I sank into the feeling of being with him, holding him, and feeling incredibly connected to him before my mind slipped into nothingness. When I came to, I wondered whether I'd fallen asleep, because I had no memory of where I had gone, and yet I was still hypnotized, sitting cross-legged with Dillon on my lap.

Now, however, he was turned around so that his back was next to my chest as he looked down at something on his lap. I leaned forward to look over his shoulder to see what had his attention. He was looking at a book.

It was closed so that I could see the cover. The dark blue background reminded me of photos taken deep in the universe, where stars are born. The intense dark blue was in the center of the cover, and as it approached the edges, it faded to a lighter blue. The letters looked as though they were a very bright, white light that seemed to illuminate so that the edges of the letters were not clearly defined. The light spelled out *Angel Babies*. It was amazingly beautiful. Startled, my eyes flew open.

A few days later, I wondered whether I could have yet another extraordinary experience with Dillon. Was it luck that allowed it to happen before? Was it all a product of my imagination? I found a comfortable place to relax and put myself in hypnosis again.

And again I deepened the trance by going down in an elevator, and when its doors opened, Dillon was standing there. As I bent down, he greeted me by taking my head in his hands and putting his face up to mine, saying firmly, "Let go of the doubt. *Let go of the doubt!* It is *me!*" Astonished, my eyes popped open. I prayed for God to help me let go of the doubt that my experiences weren't real.

On another occasion, I found myself floating to Earth with Dillon, who told me to get going on writing the book. "You can do it, Mommy," he said.

As I looked to my right, my parents were there, too, offering support and encouragement. I wrote for the next five hours.

The next day, I wrote about the actual miscarriage, and it brought up all the pain I'd felt at the time. I allowed myself to feel the sadness once again, and as I cried, I thought of the psychic saying I had a sister in spirit, whom I assumed was one of my mother's miscarriages. I called out to her to console me. The phone rang, startling me. Although I wouldn't typically pick up the phone while crying, I somehow knew that whoever was on the end of the phone line was being sent to me.

"Hello?" I said pretending to be cheerful. No one answered. "Hello?" I repeated. I could tell there was no one on the phone line. I understood the call to mean that my sister in spirit, whoever she was, was there indeed.

A couple of weeks later, I used self-hypnosis again, still visualizing an elevator slowly descending. When I reached the bottom floor, the doors opened and Dillon greeted me, along with my mom and dad, who were behind him to my right. Then I saw someone I'd never seen before. She looked to be in her early to mid-twenties, with long, blonde, silky hair and big, beautiful blue eyes. Although she was younger than I am, she felt older and looked familiar. As I scanned her features, I realized she looked like Meghan, or how Meghan would look as a grown-up. As I looked into her eyes, I somehow knew she was my sister.

They were pleased I'd heard all their messages and congratulated me on the book, telling me it was going well. I thanked them for their help. "Don't worry about Meghan," my dad assured me, "she'll be fine." Dillon said the same. Hearing their reassurances felt comforting.

They told me they were very proud of Tim. "I like him a lot," my mom said. I liked hearing that since she had passed away before they had a chance to meet.

When it was time for them to go, Dillon grinned before turning away and yelling over his shoulder, "Good-bye, Love-Love."

Amazed at the coincidence, I yelled after him, "Hey, Meghan calls me that!"

He replied, "I know. How do you think she thought of it?"

"Why are there two loves?" I asked.

"Because one is from me," he shouted back to me.

It's hard to believe now, but even after those profound experiences, I still doubted their reality. Doubt entered whenever my conscious mind got involved, and I'd wonder again about whether these things could really be happening. Although the letters I was receiving from other families who'd lost babies did provide some validation for me, I still needed to know my experiences were real. I still looked for proof, for some evidence. I didn't know why I still doubted when the other families sounded as if they absolutely believed their experiences.

By now it had become common for me to talk to my parents and Dillon any time I got a massage. I'd begin by visualizing the pool deck of the familiar Jamaican home, and as always, it was wonderful to see my parents. On one occasion, after I'd glanced away briefly, I looked back to them and found myself in another scene. Sitting before me was a young man in his early twenties. As I looked at him, I recognized it was Dillon, no longer a little boy but a young man who seemed much wiser than his years. He told me he was proud of me and my work on the book. I let his words of pride melt into me. Then, somewhat embarrassed, I glanced down. When I looked up again, there were forms standing behind him. Initially I had a hard time understanding what I was seeing, but then I became aware the forms were spirits.

As I looked behind and above Dillon, I saw different forms. Somehow I knew they were my dad, my grandfather, and my great-grandfathers. Above them were more forms that I understood to be my mother, grandmother, and great-grandmothers. They formed an inverted pyramid, with Dillon at the bottom. As I looked past the pyramid to the sides, I saw many small white wisps of moving light. I was in awe as I watched them come toward me.

Dillon sensed my puzzlement and told me, "They are the lost babies. They've come to thank you for giving them a voice." As he spoke, I watched the tiny wisps of light and let the meaning of his words take hold. A lump formed in my throat as I felt their love. I seemed to recognize some of the wisps from the stories of lost babies I had received. The feeling was so overwhelming that I fought not to start sobbing.

As the scene faded, I said urgently, "I'm sorry, Dillon. This is all incredible, but could you please show me a physical sign so that I know everything that has happened isn't a figment of my imagination? I need some kind of physical validation. I'm so sorry, but I need proof."

Suddenly, the scene changed, and I was in a gym watching a red ball rolling from one side of the floor to the other. As I looked to the right, I saw my nephew Conor. As the ball rolled to him, he kicked it into the air. I watched as the red ball sailed in the air.

"Look for the red ball," Dillon said.

When the massage ended, I dressed quickly and almost ran out to my car to search for a pen and paper to write down Dillon's message. "Look for the red ball," I said aloud as I wrote each word.

As I drove home, I imagined how I might see the red ball. Perhaps on a playground or in a store, but it didn't appear to me the way I expected. The next night, I had a dream of being in a gym. I watched as a white ball with large red hexagons rolled on the gym floor from the left to the right. I stood watching as an observer, not emotionally involved in the scene. Then the ball was kicked and began sailing through the air. With the ball in midair, I suddenly realized it was the same scene Dillon had shown me, and I became excited. "It's the ball! It's the ball!" I screamed in my inner mind before realizing I was in a dream. With that awareness, I awoke. It was morning.

I still felt the excitement of seeing the ball. It was the confirmation I had asked for, or was it? As I became more alert, I reminded myself that it was, after all, a dream. Even though I knew those on the other side could communicate with us in dreams and had before, I began to question the dream's validity. If Dillon was going to show me a ball, why didn't he show me the same red ball instead of a white one with large red hexagons on it? Why did he leave room for me to doubt?

Tim and I sat on our back porch as I told him about my dream and questioned its authenticity. Getting ready for a run, he tied his shoes as he listened to me.

Tim looked at me quizzically. "Do you still doubt this? Doesn't white mean spirituality?" he asked as he stood up to leave. "Maybe you need a little more faith," he advised as he walked down the stairs.

My jaw dropped, and my eyes popped open. *He's telling me to believe?* Stunned by his response, I sat looking at Dillon's tree for several minutes, taking in Tim's words.

I took a deep breath. "I'm so sorry, Dillon, but I still need something more. Something more tangible," I sputtered out loud. "I'm driving myself nuts with doubts."

Feeling sad that I lacked the faith Tim talked about, I walked to Dillon's tree and wrapped my arms around the trunk to hug it. *If only the tree could hold me,* I thought. My eyes fell to where a broken branch stub had prohibited me from sitting in the limbs in the past. The stub was gone. I looked on the ground to see whether it had fallen off. It had been there just two days earlier. In its place was a round opening, two inches in diameter, that looked reddish inside where the pulp was. It still felt damp, as though it had just happened. I wondered whether Tim somehow yanked it off when he was doing yard work the day before.

It didn't matter. My secret wish had been granted. I climbed into the tree. It was amazingly comfortable. Kylie and Meghan soon discovered my nest and climbed up to join me. We stayed in the tree until Tim got back from his run. "Tim, come join us in Dillon's tree," I shouted as he walked towards us.

I pointed to the hole where the stub was. It was already becoming duller in color. "Did you remove the branch stub?" I asked him.

"No, honey, I didn't."

"I think Dillon just removed it for me," I remarked.

"Wow! Well, I didn't touch it, honey," Tim added.

The next day I was to meet a girlfriend, Nancy, for coffee. While driving to her house and waiting for a traffic light to change, my thoughts went to Dillon and the red ball. Although it had been only a couple of days since Dillon had told me to look for the red ball, I hadn't seen an actual red ball, and I was exhausting myself with doubt.

Frustrated, I began a one-way conversation with Dillon in my mind. "Look, I know my dream was probably the real thing with the ball," I started, "but actually I don't know that at all. I'm so sorry, Dillon, but I need something tangible. I'm tired of questioning everything, and I'm tired of doubting. This time, I'll choose the sign. If you show me this sign, I promise you I will fully believe everything that has happened once and for all," I announced with conviction.

The word *key* came to mind. "Okay, Dillon, anything with a key. Mention a key or say the word key or whatever," I said, frustrated, "but something with a key." Nancy was a psychic. Surely she'd see him hanging over my shoulder with a key in his hand even though I had no intention of bringing it up to her. Suddenly, an antique key popped into my mind's eye. "Okay, an antique key. That's the sign."

Although Nancy and I talked for hours, neither Dillon nor a key ever came up.

The next morning, Tim and I had an appointment with Kenn, a psychic we had seen years before. Though we looked forward to it, we had nothing particular in mind. During our drive, we caught up on the current news about school, the girls, and other family matters. Talking without being interrupted was a luxury. Oddly, considering where we were going, my talk with Dillon about a key had slipped my mind, and I didn't mention it to Tim.

Once inside Kenn's home, Tim motioned for me to sit down across from Kenn and go first. As Kenn talked, he told me periodically to shuffle the cards and choose cards from different stacks. He emphatically stated they were not tarot cards but cards from England, his tone indicating his were better. I wouldn't have known the difference or cared, but it seemed important for him to tell me. As he turned over a card, he paused and asked, "Who's Maggie?"

I looked at Tim with wide eyes. "Meggie?" I restated, making sure I said the name correctly. Kenn nodded his head up and down.

"Meggie is our daughter," I answered.

Kenn continued, turning over individual cards and giving us their meaning and how they might apply to our lives. After a few minutes, he turned over a card that caused me to gasp and slam into the back of my chair. I looked at Kenn and then at Tim with wide eyes as I held my breath, trying to take in the image on the card. It was an antique key, the same antique key I'd seen in my mind's eye at the stoplight. I looked down at the symbol on the card again and exhaled. I knew my reaction was odd to them, but how could they know the card's importance to me?

"The meaning of this card," Kenn said, looking me squarely in the eyes, "is opening new doors."

I waited until the reading was over before sharing with Tim and Kenn my stoplight conversation with Dillon.

Six days later marked the five-year anniversary of hearing Dillon for the first time. I could still hear his words as they echoed in my head: *"I'm right here. I'm right* here!" Finally, and with great relief, my prayers were answered. I stopped doubting.

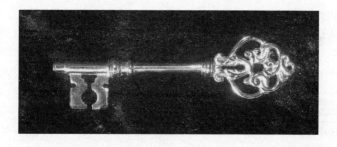

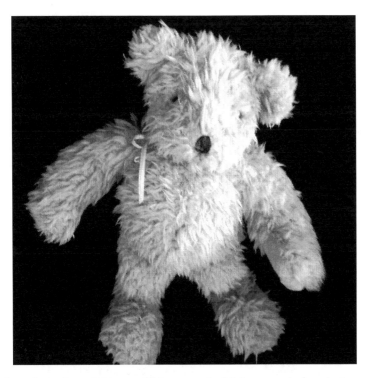

The bear I purchased for myself that matched Maryanne's description of the bear she saw in Dillon's wagon.

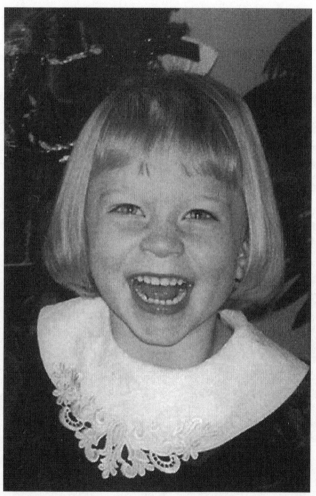

Meghan as she looked when Kenn described her as looking like a drawing on a Christmas card he had. Maryanne's description of Dillon being a towhead with big blue eyes also resembled Meghan.

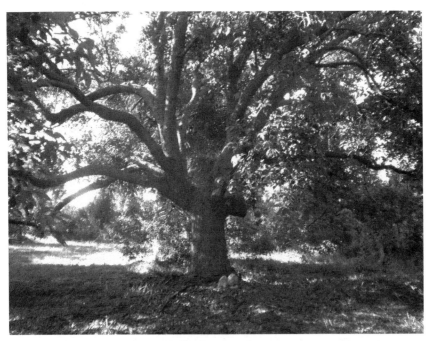

Dillon's tree today.

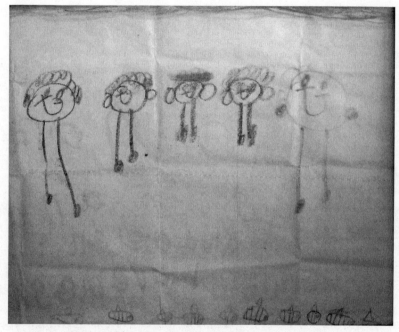

Meghan's family portrait with Dillon in the center.

HEARING FROM OUR BABIES

It was time to review all the personal stories I had received as a result of my letters published in magazines and prepare them for publication in *Angel Babies*. Although many of the people contributing their experiences gave me permission to use their full names, for the sake of privacy, I have chosen to use only their first names, and I use pseudonyms for those who requested anonymity. But the experiences related in the stories are theirs, as written to me.

While often sad, their stories are also full of acceptance, faith, and hope for the future. Some of the women haven't told their stories to anyone else or only to their husbands. They kept this information close to their hearts because of their fear of others thinking they had lost their minds. Others were quite open about their experiences and share their stories freely. I thank all of these people for their courage in sharing their personal, profound, and touching experiences of their babies. When I asked for their permission to include their stories in my book, they responded almost unanimously with a similar sentiment: If it will help other women to heal, to know they aren't alone or going crazy, or that they didn't imagine it or make it up, then yes, please share my story. That was their reason, and it is my purpose in writing this book. The real names of the babies are used, if they were named, to honor them.

The stories reveal that our babies can begin to communicate with us from before conception, throughout pregnancy, and after their passing to the other side. Their messages can come in dreams and in a half-asleep, half-awake twilight state, as well as during meditation or while in a hypnotic state. Messages have come through psychics and during near-death experiences, or by actually hearing the babies' voices or seeing them. The babies choose many means of communication, including a subtle sense of presence or through a coincidence or series of coincidences.

Communication experiences often reveal the baby's gender and other information, while some experiences seem to be preparing the mother that the baby will leave. Often when we don't understand from where the information originated, we begin to analyze and sometimes doubt the validity of our experience. We rationalize, thinking, *That can't be real*, or asking where that feeling or thought came from, or attributing the experience to our fears or imagination. We can talk ourselves out of the experience and shut off any possible communication if we allow skepticism and doubt to deny us our spiritual potential. But if we remain open and receptive to possibilities, I believe we are all capable of such experiences.

Messages in Dreams

Dreams are one of the most common ways to hear from the other side. It is in this state that many contacts have been made, because when our conscious mind is resting, our conscious defenses are down.

While dream visitations don't erase grief, they often leave the dreamers feeling more secure knowing their loved ones live on. Comforted by that knowledge, they feel more at peace.

Dream visitations stand out from other dreams in that they seem to be actual meetings. The dreamer feels it was not an ordinary or typical dream but an actual encounter. Sometimes dream visits involve telepathy, where no words are spoken, or they may involve vivid color. Dreams of those who have passed on are usually remembered clearly because of their meaning or significance to the dreamer and the profound emotions they stir. It's a time when we can once again, for even just a few brief moments, see, hear, and embrace our departed loved ones.

I believe such dreams seem real because they are actual visits or encounters rather than dreams. Our loved ones often appear as we knew them, but without any of the health problems they may have suffered from during their lives.

During a pre-birth communication the babies sometimes reveal they won't be coming. Sometimes an explanation might be given, but many times it's just to say good-bye. Some call these premonitions, the soul knowing and preparing the dreamer for what is going to happen. Other dreams can occur after the child has left the mother.

Mary wrote to me from Canada about a dream of her miscarried son, Ravine, who came to tell his mother that he still exists and is still around and that she will have a daughter

Mary and Baby Ravine

This dream occurred about a year after I miscarried my son. I always had a feeling this baby was a boy, but I couldn't be sure. My husband always had that feeling, too. The dream seemed to be about the future because I dreamt not only of the baby I'd lost, but also of the daughter I have now. In the dream, we were at my ten-year high school reunion,which we never actually attended, but I believe the reunion gave me an indication of the future time period I was looking at.

In the dream, I was sitting on the floor. We had a son around the age of two, who looked almost exactly like my husband did as a boy, with bright blonde hair and the same features. I was struck by how much he looked like my husband, Kim. My daughter, whom we had not yet had, was also there and was about nine months old. We were sitting in a circle of chairs with other old classmates of mine and their families. Ravine (our son we miscarried) was being a normal little boy, not saying much, but playing, running around, and leaning on Kim's knees. He was very attached to his papa.

I remember watching him, and though at the time I didn't realize who he was, I felt very drawn to him and had an aching to hold him. I remember wanting to stay asleep, knowing I was dreaming. Even though my daughter was in the dream (again, I didn't know her at this point), I didn't have the same feelings toward her. I realized later that it was because I wasn't losing her as I was losing Ravine. I think I had a sense that she would come and I would be able to raise her.

When I woke up, I felt a deep sense of longing, loss, and sorrow. It was a physical suffering that I didn't quite understand at that time. It took me several days to get over this feeling.

I brooded over the dream, trying to understand what it was about. Later, I came to understand it. I knew that this boy was my Ravine, and perhaps his coming to me in the dream was to reinforce to me that he is still here, that he still exists, and that he is often present. I have a strong feeling he was present at my daughter Sinead's birth.

An interesting aside is that my sister, whom I have not been very close to in the past but have been growing closer to in the last few years, also dreamt about Ravine, after Sinead was a few months old. My sister described seeing Ravine as a little boy, around three or four, who was the spitting image of Kim. I was really taken aback by that as I hadn't really discussed my miscarriage with her and hadn't told her about my dream or Ravine's face. It further reinforced to me that this is our son.

We have selectively told others about it, and most responses have been positive. When I miscarried, of course, responses were something like "Oh, it was better this way." Many people don't seem to see the baby as being a real person. But most people I have told about this experience have been very positive, and it has brought some comfort to those who have gone through miscarriages themselves.

I haven't had an experience with Ravine since that dream, and I would like to again, but I know if I don't, there is a reason, and I can accept that. I still miss him and know I will never completely get over losing him, but I don't think I should do so. The dream experience has brought me peace of mind.

A young couple from Sweden, Sarah and her husband, Anders, wrote to tell of their premonition dreams about their baby Emilie.

Sarah, Anders and Baby Emilie

My name is Sarah, and I am twenty-six years old. I live in Sweden with my husband, Anders, who is twenty-five. It was my first pregnancy, and I was almost at sixteen weeks [when the miscarriage occurred]. It has been a terrible loss in our lives since we were actively trying for a baby and very much looking forward to the birth and life ahead. The experiences we have had, though, have somehow brought comfort to what is an otherwise heartbreaking period in our lives.

We had two experiences, one before and one during the pregnancy, which I think could be categorized as being pre-birth experiences, although I have only just discovered that such things exist.

It was before the pregnancy that I had my quite straightforward experience. I had a dream one night, about three months into the time that I was actively trying to get pregnant, that my grandmother, who has been dead for ten years, appeared holding a newborn baby girl. "It'll happen," said my grandmother. "You must be patient."

I woke feeling full of confidence and no longer feeling as stressed about the whole "trying to get pregnant" issue. About two months later, we found we were expecting our first baby, and I had a feeling from the very start that the child was a girl.

Then my husband had a dream about a week before I had the miscarriage. I remember very clearly what he told me initially, that he had had a really strange dream that the baby had turned into a very beautiful butterfly and flown away. At the time, I thought nothing of it, except that it was odd that he was sharing a dream with me, which he ordinarily never does.

Anders wrote: I dreamt that my wife and I were traveling around to different types of shows, to display our big, pretty butterfly. We always received first prize when people saw our butterfly, but they were even more surprised when they saw it fly (believing it was dead and mounted, like those in museums).

But when traveling to the last show, we had a really hard time finding the place, and when we finally got there, it was packed with people who had heard of our butterfly. The place looked sort of like a church with rows of benches. When we showed our butterfly, they were all amazed. But I felt something was wrong, and the butterfly started flying higher and higher until it vanished up beyond the roof.

I was really sad that it was gone, and then I woke up. After the dream (the same night, while half-asleep), it felt like our unborn baby was the butterfly. I do not know why. It made me feel a bit sad and uneasy, but I paid no attention to it and went back to sleep. For some reason, I slept very well the rest of the night, but when I woke up and remembered the dream, I once again got the same sad and uneasy feeling.

I remember telling my wife about the dream because I thought it was odd that I remembered the dream at all. I hardly ever remember dreams, even the day after dreaming them, but this one I remembered so clearly.

Sarah continued: It wasn't until we went to the ER early in the morning of January 7, after discovering I was bleeding, that we were told that the baby had no movement or heartbeat, and it seemed from its size that it had died about a week earlier. A few days later, I remembered Anders's dream and wondered if it were mere coincidence that he had had it at the time that the baby had died inside me.

Although dreams are often symbolic in nature, we often have a sense of knowing or understanding of their deeper meaning. Here's Debbie's story of her baby boy.

Debbie and Baby Boy

In November 1996, I was inseminated with my husband's sperm, and I had six eggs implanted. I got pregnant and six weeks later learned I was carrying twins. Two weeks after that, I had a dream of two cars, one with a broken headlight.

In a separate dream, one of the babies said he had to leave because there wasn't enough for him. (I had to give myself shots to thin the blood, since I had lost two pregnancies earlier and had the lupus anticoagulant—so I believe there wasn't enough medicine for both to survive.) I then lost one of the babies. I was sad but had a bed-rest pregnancy, so everything was focused on getting the other baby here. I delivered a beautiful, healthy baby boy in August 1997.

I will always believe that the baby who left gave his life so our son Cole could live. And what a miracle he is! I will always remember his twin, even if I'm the only one, but I know, because I'm the mommy. I don't have other visions or dreams of the two other babies I lost, but they will always be a part of me. God is so good!

In the next story, Phaedra describes a male voice that came to her in a dream when she was twenty-two years old to tell her that her baby girl would not live. The voice prepared her for what was to come. Now sixty-five and living in Arizona, she relates that the male voice came to her during the most traumatic years of her life.

Phaedra and Baby Girl

In 1959, while overseas in Germany, I lost a baby in the sixth month of pregnancy. I was told by a male voice in a dream that the baby was a girl and that she would not live because she weighed only two pounds.

The next month, after delivering the baby stillborn, I heard a doctor say that that it weighed only two pounds and that it would not have survived anyway. The doctor never told me the sex of the baby; my husband told them not to tell me.

Knowing the baby would die helped me in that I already knew that something was very wrong with the pregnancy. I had lost all the fluid from the womb, and the baby had stopped moving.

The male voice was familiar to me since he had come to me before. His Biblical language was more pronounced at times, such as when I was pregnant with my last child. He said, "This child shall have many infections and be much set upon by other youth." This was very true of my last child, who just turned thirty.

Later in my life, I began reading every book on the psychiatry shelf in the library to check on whether I was really insane to have such experiences. Then I went to the next shelf and read every book in the paranormal section. I learned that there were other people like me, and I was quite relieved.

Lee, a law school student, wrote to me from Southern California. She reveals many experiences of being contacted by her baby boy, Kyler, including in a dream and through a psychic, as well as by feeling his mischievous tug and finding items moved around.

Lee and Baby Kyler

I actually hesitated to write and finally decided that if what happened to me gives comfort to just one person who went through anything similar, it will have been worth it.

When I was about six months pregnant, I had a wonderful dream. I dreamt that I was out of my body, kind of hovering over myself as I slept. In my dream, I could see inside my stomach. I saw my baby boy all curled up in the fetal position and the most beautiful angel with gold wings sitting on top of my stomach. I have never had a dream where I saw an angel before, and never had an out-of-body experience. It was incredible. I could see the angel's chest inflating as he breathed; it seemed so real. As I was looking at the baby sleeping inside me the angel started talking to me, telling me not to worry and that everything was going to be okay. I woke up the next morning with an awesome sense of peace and tranquility. During the whole pregnancy, I had had a hard time keeping food down and would throw up between six and twelve times a day. That had worried me, but with this experience, all my fears were laid to rest. The real meaning of this dream didn't become clear until much later.

It was in June 2001, on the day of my seven-month check up. I was excited because I had a surprise baby shower thrown for me at work, and my husband and I had just bought a new house to have more room for our first child. Kevin came with me to the appointment. He was supposed to have jury duty that day, but for some strange reason, he was told too many people had been called, and he was sent home. He was completely elated because he had wanted to be able to go to the doctor with me. In retrospect, I believe it was divine intervention that he was there.

The doctor checked the heartbeat and took longer than usual. I nervously joked with him that he better hurry up and find the heartbeat because he was starting to scare me. He informed me that maybe something was wrong with his machine and that they were going to give me an ultrasound. I hadn't panicked yet but was starting to feel that tightness in my throat and burning in my eyes one gets when trying to hold back tears. He gave me the ultrasound and saw that there was no heartbeat and that the baby was dead. I instantly started to cry, not just a little, but so hard that I even hyperventilated and began to shake. They got me a bag to breathe into. They informed me that the safest way for this problem to be solved was to put me through labor. Because I was only twenty-one and this was my first child, they didn't want to give me a Caesarian. They told me to go home, eat something, and come back, and by then a hospital room would be ready for me. The next thirty-six hours were the worst hours of my life. I thought I had been through hard times before, but they were nothing compared to this.

The labor took thirty-six hours because my cervix was not soft, and it took forever for them to try a number of different things to get me dilated. I told them I didn't want to be drugged because I wanted to be able to remember the experience, but I wouldn't have wished it on my worst enemy. The birth itself seemed to happen almost in slow motion. I was able to feel the head come out, then the shoulders, and finally the rest. I was crying the entire time as I had never cried before. The birth itself was a beautiful, surreal experience despite everything else that was happening at the same time. Just to think that God makes our bodies capable of something like that!

I never knew you could love something so much that you had never physically touched before. I have a very supportive husband, who was there along with other family members, but nothing anyone said made me feel better. When the doctor was asking what food I wanted and whether he could do anything else, I lashed out at him, saying, "Yeah, you could make him alive." I felt bad later for saying that. They found that the baby had been dead inside of me for about two weeks because of a knot in the umbilical cord that had cut off all nutrients. That led them to believe I could have some sort of serious infection. They took twenty vials of blood from me, testing each with everything they could to make sure I was okay and nothing else had caused Kyler's death. By the grace of God, the tests came back negative. Thankfully, the doctors said I was fine and so was my husband, and we could try again any time we felt like it.

When I got home from the hospital, I didn't leave my house to go anywhere for about three weeks. I was in an utter state of shock, depression, anger, and sadness. I think I cried myself to sleep for the first week. All my husband could do was hold me, and he also cried sometimes. Men and women grieve very differently. If you're not careful to respect and support what the other spouse is going through, something like this experience could tear apart even a strong marriage.

That was the first blow. The second happened a month later, when my husband was laid off. He's a computer programmer and lost his job when the dot-com bubble burst. After that, 9/11 happened, and the economy was shot. He was out of work for ten months. We got to the point where we were putting groceries on our credit card. I often thought, *Dear God, what have I done to deserve this?* Everything I had wanted with all my heart in the last year was falling to pieces. I hated life, I hated living, I hated feeling my pain, and each day I felt like I was just going through the motions, not really being part of any of it. We realized we had to sell our house. All through these times, the grace of God was shown, though I didn't always want to recognize it. We didn't know how we were going to make our next mortgage payment, but three days after we put our house on the market, it sold. That's almost unheard of. It had to have been divine intervention.

My in-laws are wonderful, kindhearted people, and they let us move in until we could get back on our feet. They lived far away from where I worked, and I had to quit my job. I was never the praying kind, but my mom had brought me up in a spiritual environment. I have to say, I started to pray. I was praying for anything: hope for the future, hope that things would get better. I just wanted something to go right.

My mom had a well-known friend who does psychic readings, and for some comfort, I contacted her to see what she had to say. I got an interesting message from her, part of which I understand, and part of which I may never understand, but it's interesting nonetheless. She told me that Kyler was around me from time to time, and I just had to get over some of my own limitations to feel it. She told me that he had been sent for a very important reason and that it is something I chose to do as a life path before I was even born. She said Kyler was sent to me to heal seven generations past, and seven generations to come. I have never figured out the past part, but the future part is crystal clear.

My father and I had never had a close relationship until then. My parents divorced when I was nine, and I hardly ever saw him or talked to him when I was between the ages of thirteen and nineteen. When I moved back to California at nineteen, we tried to have a relationship but ran into a lot of bumps along the way. He had never really been there for me. But when I was admitted to the hospital, my father came as soon as he could. He was in the hospital the entire time and didn't leave once, not even to get food. He had others bring it to him. When I was going through the labor, my father was holding one hand, and my husband was holding my other hand. More healing took place in those thirty-six hours than could have taken place in ten years. Once again, I feel that it was divine intervention working through the spirit of Kyler.

Soon after we moved into my in-laws' house, my husband found a wonderful job. I decided that instead of going back to work, I would go back to school; he was making enough money to allow me to do that. We have since come full circle. We now own a brand-new two-story house in Southern California, and I have been accepted to law school. I'm working part-time in a law firm and will start law school in August.

There was one day in particular when I was feeling sad thinking about Kyler and all that had happened. Just as I was about to cry, I felt a tug on my backpack, almost as if someone had pulled me back. I turned around, but no one was there. I then looked at my backpack and noticed it was unzipped. I am under the impression that Kyler is a playful, mischievous, childlike soul.

Another incident happened in my in-laws' store. They have a gift shop that sells only angels. Every night, they put everything back in place and turn off all the lights. They have to do that or the alarm won't work right when they close the door. Well, they came in one day, which just happened to be a day I was going to help them, to find some of the lights on, which they knew they had turned off. Some of the items they had put on a shelf were now on the floor, nowhere near the shelf they had been on. I am under the impression that this was Kyler, just letting me know he's around now and that he just wanted to say hi.

Even though it's been almost two years, it's still hard sometimes. When one of my friends gets pregnant or when I see a little boy about two, sometimes my mind wanders, and I think about what might have been. Then I remember that there is hope and everything happens for a reason, even if we don't understand it all the time. They say time heals all pain. I don't believe that. I believe that time makes it easier to cope, and time helps you learn how to become a better, stronger person with more character.

My husband and I are now in a better place to start a family when we feel ready. These things have brought us closer together and escalated our love for each other to a level I didn't think was imaginable. You never know how strong you are until bad things happen, and you never realize how much you need to rely on faith and hope until you have nothing else to go on. No matter how dark the situation seems, it will get better, and there is a brighter day ahead. I thought when I had the dream I described earlier that it meant everything was going to be fine with the pregnancy. I now know that it really meant that no matter what happens in life, everything will eventually turn out fine.

As you've read, I have been to hell and back in the last two years, but if telling my story can touch just one person and make her believe she can get through it and that things will get better, it will have been worth it.

Just as losing a child can test our faith, it can also cause us to doubt ourselves and wonder what we did or didn't do that might have caused the baby not to come. Understanding that it wasn't our fault can bring great peace, as Lisa's story of her son Walter illustrates.

Lisa and Baby Walter

Our son Walter, my first child, was stillborn in February 2001, when I was twenty weeks pregnant with him. The doctor who helped us through the delivery believed he died around fifteen weeks' gestation. My husband and I didn't know he had died until I was nineteen weeks pregnant. The week between knowing and delivering was surreal. I felt like a walking tomb.

The day after the delivery, I had a vivid dream about a boy who was two or three years old. He was standing under a shelter by a lake, wearing a life jacket. The jacket wasn't buckled and cinched right. I fastened it for him so he'd be safe. Then I gave him a big hug. His parents were sitting nearby. I told them my son had just died.

I'll never know for sure whether the boy in this dream was my son, but whoever he was, I believe he came to me so I would let go of trying to figure out what had caused my son to die and wondering if it was somehow my fault. You see, the dream indicates that he wasn't my child to save. He belonged to someone, or maybe something, else.

Gwen wrote to me from the southwestern United States about her dream of seeing an infant boy who wanted to come to her but was born later to another mother.

Gwen and Baby Boy

I was very touched by your research on lost babies because I believe mine contacted me through a dream. I have never told anyone about it, not even my husband. I hope you won't mind that I don't give my real name. I am still not over my actions at the time and probably never will be.

Nearly twenty-five years ago, at our "advanced" ages of forty-two and forty-six, my husband and I found ourselves expecting another child.

Quite frankly, we were not willing to have another one. Our youngest child was already eighteen years old and had just graduated high school. Two others were in college. The oldest was married with a baby of her own. My career was taking off; I had been promoted to management the year before. My husband had retired for health reasons, and we really didn't know what sort of life expectancy he had to look forward to. (As it turned out, he died ten years later.) We were nearly finished raising our children and looking forward to more grandchildren. You get the picture, I'm sure.

At about eight weeks, my pregnancy was terminated. I grieved all the same. Whatever option a woman chooses when faced with an unwanted pregnancy, there are consequences she must live with for the rest of her life.

A few months later, I had a rather vivid dream in which I seemed to be at a party. Across a very crowded room, I saw a baby about six months old, dressed for bed in those sweet snap-together pajamas, long-sleeved and footed. I rushed over to him, knowing somehow it was a baby boy. I held him and said, "Oh, you've been born!" I was very happy for that. And he replied to me telepathically and rather sadly, "Yes, but I really wanted you for my mother."

Was that my child? Yes, I believe he was. Just knowing he had been born gave me some peace.

Sometimes it isn't the mother or father who receives the communication. It can come to a family member or friend, as in Phyllis's case. Phyllis saw her friend's recently deceased husband and their two miscarried children.

Phyllis and Friend's Baby Boy and Girl

In July 1986, a very dear friend passed rather quickly back to spirit. As would be expected, his wife was beside herself with grief in the following days and weeks, her feelings magnified by her beliefs, which did not allow for communication from her husband, Frank.

One night, Frank appeared at my bed to get me up to attend his homecoming party. In the twinkling of an eye, we entered together. A cheer went up, a grand Irish shindig it was! Everyone was so grateful to see him return. It was a huge room with hundreds of people, and he started to work the room. Music and dancing, food and merriment were everywhere. Everybody I had ever heard him talk about was there, and I recognized all of them. Absolutely amazing! Among them were two children, about seven and nine; one, a girl, would not leave him alone. They danced and played around his legs, and grabbed at him relentlessly, trying to get his attention as he renewed relationships. I would not even have noticed these two if they had not been so obnoxious (to my mind). I kept looking for someone to come for them or admonish them or something, which never happened. The night wore on, and I knew I would have to leave and return to my world.

Frank did not want to hear that. "Just a few more minutes. Come meet so-and-so." He begged me to stay. I knew I couldn't do that. I still had work to do on Earth. He truly did try to persuade me, but I knew I had to go. As we came to the entrance, I realized there were many of these huge rooms here, with many parties. As I navigated the circular drive to the car, which had been provided for me, Frank and I said our farewells, and I found myself sitting on the side of my bed.

The event was so real that there was no question I had gone with Frank to his homecoming that night. It was so totally live and real! I still have only to think about it to be there again.

I arranged to see Frank's wife later that day and told her about this episode. She was stunned—and angry! I did mention these two brats (as I saw them) who never left him alone. They were ringing bells for her, because it seems she had had two miscarriages that coincided with these two children's ages. The only reason they were portrayed as brats was to get my attention, so I would specifically pass on that information and she would accept that he was fine and these children were not lost to them.

There is no question in my mind that I was allowed to participate in this wonderful event because Frank's wife needed to know he was fine, that life does indeed go on, and that love can still be communicated. These children that I could not have known about were the convincing factors for his wife.

Even the briefest dream can bring healing. Sometimes the experience is so simple that it's profound, like Holly's dream of her baby boy.

Holly and Baby Boy

After I had my first miscarriage, I had a dream. In it, I could hear the baby crying, and I knew it was a boy. I'd had a D&C that day, and so I might have still had drugs in my system, but after I woke up, I had a renewed sense of peace and felt like everything was okay.

Since my initial contact when Holly told me of her dream, she wrote to tell me that she'd given birth to twins.

Judith wrote to me from Brooklyn, New York, about delayed grieving for her lost son Adam and finally finding peace.

Judith and Baby Adam

When I was thirty-four and almost too old to be a mother, my husband and I tried to have our first child, but I had difficulty conceiving. I finally did and went to an obstetrician, but after several weeks, I began staining and had a miscarriage. The doctor never called me back, and I went through eighteen hours of pain and bleeding on my own.

Years later, now with two teenage children, I had knee problems and went to see a chiropractor who'd treated me with skill and kindness. During this process, I began to realize how much mistrust of the medical profession I had, partly because of the miscarriage experience. I also realized that I had never done the work of grieving for the lost baby that I should have done. I decided to create my own ritual in the week before Easter and read a psalm and part of a service for the dead out of a prayer book each day. Early on Easter morning, I read the last psalm and prayer and lit a candle. As I lit it, I had a clear memory of a dream I had the night before, which I had forgotten on awakening.

In the dream, I saw a little boy, about ten years old, who called himself Adam. He was a bit pudgy, had a stylishly short buzz-cut hairdo, and was wearing a white, ribbed turtleneck shirt. I didn't have any feelings of love for him; in fact, he was a little too cocksure for my tastes and nothing whatsoever like my own beloved son. (It was, in fact, more than fifteen years earlier when I'd had the miscarriage, but his name had much meaning for me because I had written a poem after the miscarriage in which I had envisioned my lost baby.) The little boy did not want to leave, but he was met by his father and other relatives, who persuaded him to go with them. There was a sense of release and happiness for everyone concerned as he walked off with his father, hand in hand.

I don't usually remember dreams after I get out of bed, and since the memory came exactly as I was lighting the candle, I felt the dream was an answer to a prayer and that the spirit of the lost child who had been hovering around me was now taken up to heaven with his father from the previous life. I had no sense of recognition of the father in the dream scene where the boy meets his dead relatives, so familiar from Dr. Raymond Moody's books. [Many people in Dr. Moody's books report seeing a relative who had passed on when they had near-death experiences.]

In the months after my dream, I began to see Adam in my meditations. He serves as a gatekeeper for the channeling of my dead relatives, with his own insistent ritual involving pink roses. I did such meditations only a few times because they were so tiring, but I felt Adam was an enabling and protective presence. Were I to attempt anything like that now (about five years later), I feel sure Adam would still be there for me.

Erin wrote from Australia with a dream experience about her twins, Sarrah and Taliah, that would continue on and off throughout the night and gave her closure. She also received answers to her questioning whether it was her fault one of the babies had died and whether the baby forgave her. Here is Erin's story.

Erin and Baby Sarrah

I was pregnant with twins, Taliah and Sarrah, and lost one, Sarrah, at nineteen weeks' gestation due to a horrible condition called Twin-to-Twin Transfusion Syndrome (TTTS). The babies start out healthy and normal, but due to a problem in the placenta causing incorrect blood flow between the twins, it leads to the death of one or both. Once one of the twins dies, the syndrome is over.

I had dreams several weeks after she died, after I had gone through the shock and the denial stage of grief. The dreams were all on the same night, but they were separate because I woke after each one, got up, had a drink, went to the bathroom, and then went back to sleep. Then I would have the next dream.

In my first dream, I was in an operating theatre, and they delivered both girls by C-section. One was okay while the other had a team of medical people working on her for ages, and in the end, they stopped and said there was nothing more they could do. She never took a breath of life, and it was a very difficult time for me.

My second dream seemed to start where the first one had finished, as if the message wasn't completed yet. It was after the delivery; everyone was looking at Taliah, and Sarrah was alone. I went over to Sarrah and looked at her tiny body, lifeless and still. I wanted her to know that I loved her, and so I wrapped her in a baby blanket. She opened her eyes and smiled at me. It was as if she understood that I loved her, but she couldn't stay. When she opened her eyes, there was something about the expression on her face, like she was very weak and frail. Something was wrong with her.

Then I had the third dream. We were out as a family, and I was carrying a beautiful little girl. She was about three years old, with long, blonde, wavy hair, blue eyes, and gorgeous skin. In my heart, I felt it was Sarrah. I felt like I never wanted to put her down. My husband was carrying Taliah, and our other children were walking with us. This dream had such a warm feeling accompanying it.

In fact, all these dreams were accompanied by a warm feeling, and they were in color. I usually dream in black and white, and I don't usually see faces. I saw Sarrah several times. I can still sense her, and I feel she is just waiting for the right time. She sings to me sometimes when I am in the sleep-wake phase. I wake up with a sweet song in my head that I haven't heard for many years, such as "Morning Has Broken," or "Good Morning, Starshine." Believe me, I am a hip-hop kind of a girl, and these songs are nice but not those I would think of out of the blue.

The amazing thing is, I went for a scan at twenty-one weeks and was told that one of my babies had died two weeks prior. At that time, they had no idea whether my twins were identical or fraternal. I had to carry both to thirty-eight weeks for the sake of the survivor. So I had no proof that the baby I lost was a girl or whether they were identical; I only saw it in my dreams. Also, I didn't know the cause of death before the autopsy and blamed myself terribly for the rest of the pregnancy. I asked Sarrah to show me a yellow flower if she forgave me and to show me a red flower if it wasn't my fault. When I was in the hospital having Taliah and Sarrah, the flowers I received were all red and yellow.

I used to think I was going nuts, but now I think Sarrah gave her life so that Taliah would be healthy. She knew that she had problems because of the TTTS and that her body was not well. The longer the syndrome continues, the more risk there is to both twins. The survival rate is very low for both babies without laser surgery, which wasn't available yet in Australia. I believe she stayed alive for the first ultrasound so that I could see her alive, since she died shortly after. I never felt her leave me.

I don't feel I've lost something anymore. I think about her all day, every day, but it isn't with sadness. I am just waiting for her return because I know she will come again. I don't know when exactly; I just know she will.

A writer, Jane lives on the Chesapeake Bay with her husband and two-year-old daughter. Raised Catholic, she does not practice any religion currently, saying she didn't believe in the Catholic God or in the god of any religion but does believe there is more to life than mere biology. Here is Jane's story of her baby boy.

Jane and Baby Boy

I've put off writing to you long enough. It's still kind of like scraping at a scab to think too much about it, but writing can help.

I miscarried our second child three weeks ago, at about eleven weeks along, but I had known that I would miscarry much, much longer—in fact, long before I got pregnant. There's nothing I can attribute the feeling to since I've never had a miscarriage before. I had been somewhat obsessed with miscarriage experiences for maybe a year before I got pregnant. I was obsessed in a strange way, as though I knew on some level, not too far from my consciousness, that a miscarriage would happen this time around. I've had such feelings before about other important events in my life, and I've learned to recognize them and accept them for the truth they likely are.

So, once I was pregnant, I found myself afraid to go away overnight without a huge bag of heavy pads, just in case I started bleeding. I refused to tell any friends about the pregnancy, just in case I would then have to tell them I had lost the baby.

At about eight weeks, I experienced a very short dream. I was standing somewhere, and suddenly I began to gush blood. I awakened from this dream extremely sad, and then all of a sudden was thrilled to find out it was only a dream after all.

At around eleven weeks, I was at a playground with our daughter when I felt wetness between my legs—not quite the same sensation as in the dream, but close. I touched my pants leg, and there was bright red blood on my hand. There wasn't that much, and even though I bled on and off that day, there was no real cramping. I told my husband that I might be miscarrying but that I couldn't be certain. I still had some hope.

That night, I had a short but very powerful waking dream, where I was in a half-awake state but couldn't move. In the dream, I saw a white, pure light surround my belly and my uterus for just a second. I knew it was healing light, and even though it appeared to be moving inward, I knew that the baby was gone. Seconds after the white light appeared, I saw a figure. An angel? I don't know since my religious beliefs don't include angels, but that's the only being I can relate this vision to. This figure brushed the hair from my face, and tenderly, as a mother or father would, tucked the covers up around my shoulders.

I awakened from this dream or vision knowing the miscarriage was real. Even though the bleeding was light for the next four days, every time I would think, *It's just bleeding; the baby's fine*, a feeling of truth would come over me, and I would realize once again that it was real. The cramps began with a vengeance four days later, and it was all over three days after that.

Strangely, I had a strong feeling the child was a boy. I say that because my husband and I always believed that we would have two girls. Also, I had not been able to get any sense of how he would be born or whether the birth would go well or not. Now I know why. And now that the miscarriage is over, I seem to feel a girl spirit visiting our family. Only time will tell whether she will come to us.

I have been meditating on what happened, and as I've done so, I've had a strong feeling that the boy I carried for just a few weeks wasn't really ours. We were just holding him—briefly—and he really belongs to some other family. I don't have a better explanation for this feeling. It's very hard to put into words, but I do feel that even though we had a connection to him, he wasn't ours to keep, at least not this time.

Sylvia contacted me from Puerto Rico to tell her dream of discovering she was pregnant with a girl and a later dream of learning why the baby couldn't stay.

Sylvia and Baby Girl

In a dream, I saw myself through the lens of a camera that went up inside me until I saw something added to my uterus. When I woke up, I knew I was pregnant and told my husband so. I was happy because we had been married for nine years without having children, and I wanted to be a mother.

It was a complicated time because of my father-in-law's medical condition of dementia. His illness took us by surprise, and we didn't have the money to deal with it. My husband was unemployed while waiting for his medical license, and my salary at the time wasn't enough for the three of us.

Almost three weeks later, I miscarried. That night, I had a dream where I was in a hurry to meet with my child. In the dream, I knew that she had to go, and so I had to get to the meeting place quickly. When I got there, it was a place in the open air, with trees in the background and a table like a church altar that a priest stands behind. She was there and had wings; she was flying over the table, waiting for me. I looked at her and noticed she was a girl, but at the same time, I always knew it. I noticed that she looked older, like a two-year-old child, but I didn't feel there was anything strange about it. In fact, it felt quite normal. She talked to me and said, "Mom, I'm sorry. I have to leave you. It is not a good time to come into your life right now. I love you. I will see you later."

I answered, "It's okay, baby. I understand, and I will see you later." Then I sent her a kiss, and she flew away. When I woke up, I told my husband about the dream with a happy attitude, because she came to say good-bye and she was a beautiful girl. I felt so happy that I could talk to her that I didn't feel sorry for the miscarriage. She looked so peaceful and beautiful that I didn't care about myself. I felt that if she cared enough to come to me in a dream to say good-bye, then who am I to focus on my sorrow and not feel the gratitude of the experience of love?

A month later, my husband died. The day I buried him, his medical license arrived, and I buried it with him. The past three years have been the hardest of my life, but at the same time, I feel strong and thank God for all my experiences.

Melissa Anne wrote to me from the northwestern United States about a healing dream of her lost baby, Helem.

Melissa Anne and Baby Helem

I had planned to have a gentle, natural birth with my living son, Michael. What I got was the complete opposite: two days of painful failed induction followed by a C-section and separation from my baby hours after he was born. Later, I found out that the doctor had lied to me about almost everything and that the interventions and C-section were completely unnecessary. This left me feeling very depressed and broken. The trauma around Michael's birth sent me into major postpartum depression.

When Michael was six months old, I had a dream that I believe my last miscarried baby sent me. (I have had five pregnancies, and four of them have been early miscarriages.) In my dream, I am in my bedroom, sitting on the floor next to the bed, with my knees up, as if I were doing sit-ups. It is early in the morning, and the birds are singing. I am at the pushing stage of labor. I do not look very pregnant. I push gently when I have the urge, but am letting my body do most of the work. Finally, a baby emerges, and I bring it to my chest and hold it tight. My husband is behind me, and I am leaning on him as if he were a high-back chair. He is caressing the baby and me gently with his hands. I begin to breast-feed the baby, and we never look to discover the baby's gender. It was so peaceful and beautiful, and quite healing for me—the most vivid dream I have ever had. When I woke up, I felt it had really happened. I was about one week pregnant but did not know it at the time.

When I discovered that I was pregnant, I knew right away the dream was a message from my baby, but what did it mean? Was I going to have an unassisted home birth? Was I going to miscarry, as I had before? I wanted the first to be the outcome, but it wasn't. About two weeks after the dream, I had been awake for about thirty minutes when I felt something wet; my miscarriage had begun. It was peaceful and unassisted; my body did all the work, and my husband was a tremendous support (he was behind me in the dream). It was too early to determine the gender of the baby, so we will never know. Also, this child would have been due in January. I live in Washington State, and there are not many birds here in January. I feel that this dream was my baby saying hello and telling me that everything is okay, and he knows that I love all my babies with all my heart, even if they never develop to full term.

Reflecting on the dream, it was like I was given the birth I was supposed to have. I really felt that I had been given a second chance, and I did it the way I had planned in the first place. The baby I lost gave me a peaceful, gentle, and sacred birth before it left my body. I felt renewed and healed in many ways. My depression has lifted greatly since that dream. You would expect that the loss of the child would have sunk me deeper into despair, but it did not because the baby gave me the birth I was wanting and at the same time said hello and let me know that it could feel my love for him and for all my babies, living or not.

Moreover, I had never had a dream where I connected with any of my babies, not even Michael. Once I knew I was losing this baby, I was overjoyed that I had been able to connect with him in my dream. I knew that he knew what was going to happen, and he came to me to let me know that it was okay and meant to be. None of my other babies helped me see that; even though these babies were lost quite early, they could still feel my love for them. It also gave me more than the joy of being with child for a short time, which is all I had with my previous miscarriages. I was able to hold my baby and caress him and nurse him, something that would never have happened if I had not had that dream. I kind of got to know him as he was in spirit, if that makes any sense.

My husband and I have named the baby Helem, a boy's name, although we do not know the gender of the baby. The name Helem originates in the Bible and signifies both dreaming and healing.

Later, Melissa Anne wrote to me again about the birth of a baby girl. The story illustrates how dreams can be understood on many levels.

I had a baby girl, Sarah, who was born at home, with just my husband and me there. It was the end of spring, my windows were open, and I could hear the birds singing as my labor was finishing up that morning. The birds continued to sing for us all morning as we celebrated Sarah's birth. It really was just as my dream had shown me, except that I gave birth in a portable whirlpool bath instead of on the floor. But the peaceful labor and connection with my husband and then the bond and tenderness all three of us shared after the birth were identical to my dream.

I have not had any other experiences with Helem after my miscarriage, but I feel that little spirit with me always. Sometimes I think that maybe my little girl is Helem because we have the same kind of spiritual connection, but that is something I guess I will never know for sure. Maybe Helem was a spirit sent here to let me know that I needed to prepare for Sarah because she would be with me soon, and I was meant to have an unassisted birth; or maybe it was Sarah stopping in a little early to let me know that she was on her way and she wanted to be born at home. Either way, it was Helem who helped me see how I was to give birth. The whole experience, from that dream all the way to my daughter's birth, has changed my life forever in wonderful ways.

In the next story of Ann-Marie's dream of her baby, Micah, she learns many lessons and is comforted in knowing the baby will return to her in the future.

Ann-Marie and Baby Micah

Several weeks ago, I began having some bleeding when I should have been ovulating, and after a week, I was getting worried. The first thing I did was take a pregnancy test, even though I was sure it would be a total waste of time given I hadn't had sex since before my last period. Well, it was positive. I was in shock! We had been trying, but I had given up.

Since I had been spotting for a week, I knew it was possible I could lose the baby. Within the next few days, the bleeding increased, and I experienced horrible pain. My husband was worried that it was an ectopic pregnancy, and so we went to the hospital to get it checked out.

They said it was a threatened miscarriage and that we should go home and rest and come back in a couple of days to check the HCG levels.

I tried to convince myself everything would be okay, but by Sunday night, I was losing hope. I was to get my blood tested on Monday. I knew the baby was dead and decided not to go, but later decided that I just had to know for sure. The hospital confirmed it. I also found out that I'd been two months pregnant (established by the HCG levels), not a couple of weeks.

Around this time, I started getting an idea of the baby's name. The name Michael popped out at me everywhere, but it wasn't quite right.

Three nights ago, I had a dream. The spirit of the baby came to me. We spoke no words—it was like a soul communication. I don't know whether I can explain it properly. There was just sudden knowledge, as if he were feeding information directly to my brain. It wasn't like someone telling you something and then you sort through it and figure out what was meant. This communication was knowledge, complete acceptance, and peace. He explained to me why he could not be born. I felt there was karma involved. Then he showed me what he would have looked like. He was so horribly deformed that I could not bear to look at him. I was upset that I could feel so horribly about a child who was my own, but he told me that it was okay. It was one reason he would not be born. I also suddenly knew his name: Micah.

Last night, I finally began to miscarry. My husband thinks I am grasping for a sense of connection to the baby, but the dream seemed to have such great depth to it, and the feeling about the name was strong.

Ann-Marie wrote again after several weeks, answering questions I had asked about her dream communication with Micah.

The dream came three days before the miscarriage. I wanted to know why the baby had died. This question was constantly in my mind as the days passed. I wanted to understand, but I didn't consciously go to bed looking for an answer.

Micah came to me in the form of a man, but not completely defined. The communication was mind to mind and very specific. There was a total knowing, a complete understanding of everything he told me. Nothing was left for me to figure out, which was what I felt was the gift of this communication. There was complete acceptance and peace—except when I was shown his deformity—but I wonder whether that was an emotion he felt I needed to experience, even briefly.

Basically, I had thought from the beginning there was a lesson for me, karma, as I mentioned earlier. I came to my conclusions about what it was, and Micah verified it for me and added more insights and explanations. Micah's reasons for not staying were personal, but in no way do I feel punished, although someone could possibly think that. Even as he confirmed his reasons, I absolutely knew it was a gift, if you will, to help me grow, to teach a lesson that I would not learn otherwise. It was not malicious, but it was the only way I would get it. I will say this, though: one of the reasons was to give me clarity regarding my marital situation. My miscarriage was an instant revelation on those accounts.

You see, I had told my husband I was leaving him the day before I took the pregnancy test. After the test, when I knew with certainty I was pregnant, the spotting went from brown to red, and it seemed that a miscarriage was imminent.

Once I had the dream, I felt at peace. I felt such love and beauty when Micah came to me, and I loved him more for coming to me to guide me through this. The fact that I learned his name put me even more at peace. And the peace—that was the biggest gift of all. I just know it was a powerful, awesome dream. I just hate saying "dream," though, because even as I was experiencing it, I knew it was beyond any dream.

An odd thing happened as I was typing this. I have been wondering lately whether I will ever get a chance to have children again, and I just had this feeling of a warm presence and the idea that someday I will have another child, and he will be Micah. I have to say, despite all I have read lately, I feel crazy just saying that!

Nadine wrote to me from Boston about a healing dream contact with a baby she aborted and grieved about for years.

Nadine and Baby

Three or four years after I terminated a pregnancy, I dreamt of the baby. I often thought of and mourned the baby. The dream was very healing. I think the communication was telepathic; I don't remember the exact words, if there even were any. The child was genderless and was the age mine would have been had it been born. She or he assured me that all was well and all was forgiven. It was enormously relieving to have had that contact—a big step toward my forgiving myself, as if a big weight had been lifted. It was as though I knew that the baby knew I wanted him or her and that he or she understood. Thank you for the opportunity to share.

Messages through Psychic Experiences

Many psychics can bring messages from the other side. Some psychics see visions or hear communications from departed souls. Some experience strong intuitive feelings about an individual's concerns or future events. Some use cards or objects to help them focus. Some employ more than one method in giving a reading to a subject. Messages come by different means, which are almost as individual as the psychics themselves.

A psychic healer, Jeanene Herr from Lawrenceville, Georgia, wrote about her practice.

Jeanene Herr

In my work, people from the other side often show up during my sessions. I have found they appear to me both from abortion and miscarriage. Apparently, they continue to grow or else they just show themselves to me at various ages so that I can understand the timeframe of the event. I did a session for a woman and told her she needed to forgive herself and her son. She said she did not have a son. I told her I was seeing a young man about twenty-two years old standing behind her with his hands on her shoulders and that he said he's her son. She finally admitted that twenty-two years ago, she'd had an abortion.

Psychics often let the parents know their babies are in the company of other departed loved ones. A freelance writer from Florida, Ellen shared her experience of being contacted by her baby Ariella when a family friend had a private reading through a renowned psychic medium.

Ellen and Baby Ariella

I was forty-one weeks into my first pregnancy and in the hospital, progressing very slowly through labor, when all of a sudden there was a big gush of blood. They rushed me into an emergency C-section, but our baby girl, Ariella, was already gone.

Exactly three months later, one of my husband's friends, a good friend but someone we see only every six months or so, went to visit a well-known psychic. Surprisingly, the friend came back with a message for us. The psychic had told him he had a friend who had suffered a loss, and the person's name began with M, like Mike or Mark. Well, not exactly, but my husband's name is Manny. Then he said the mother's name was Ellen. It was a child, and the loss had something to do with blood (Ariella bled to death). The child wanted them to know she was okay and that she was with Ellen's side of the family, someone with a G or a J. My mother, Gertrude, had just passed away in April of that same year.

I was stunned, but at the same time, not surprised at all. There was this sense that it was true. There was also my skeptical mind, which kept telling me there must be some trick to it. That was the beginning of a spiritual journey for my husband and me. I used to question life after death. Today, I have no questions.

Several years after sharing her story with me, Ellen wrote again.

The other day, I was at a healing circle, and a woman came up to me and asked whether I worked with my little girl guide. She told me, "She's about eight years old, looks just like you, and I think her name is something like Ellie." Well, Ariella would be eight, and I have really had no feeling of a connection with her—until now. I feel we have reconnected, and then your letter arrived right after. So the story goes on. I know your book will be very healing for many, many people. I'm proud to be part of it.

Energies often come through to the psychic when spirits know someone can pass on the message to a loved one. Daniel tells about his experience with his babies, Jesse and Samuel, coming through to relatives in a group experience and again in a private reading with noted psychic medium George Anderson. In addition to Jesse and Samuel, other departed loved ones within his and his wife's families, including babies Brian and Sarah, came through as well.

Daniel and Babies Jesse, Samuel, Brian and Sarah

My wife and I were married for more than five years before we tried to have children. The first pregnancy ended in miscarriage, and the second pregnancy resulted in a premature birth at about twenty-eight weeks. The baby's main problem was that his lungs were too premature, and he was dependent on a respirator for oxygen. His brief life had a major impact on our lives.

My son Jesse lived for sixteen days. During this roller coaster period of many ups and downs between life and death, my wife Margaret and I hung in with him in every way we could, until the end. I come from a large family, and we love children. Some of my siblings and spouses had come from other states to visit during Jesse's stay in the hospital and offer support. Virtually all of them made the trip to attend the funeral on short notice. After the funeral, they went to a local nursery, bought a large ornamental cherry tree, and planted it in our front yard in Jesse's memory. We've since moved to another house in a different town, but we still go back from time to time to see the tree. It's particularly beautiful in the spring.

In addition, my mother and one of my sisters started a scholarship fund in Jesse's name. My wife and I maintain it, and it has been used to give modest scholarships to each of Jesse's cousins (he has a lot of them) to congratulate them on reaching their first year of college. Perhaps it will also extend to help their children when they come of age.

Losing Jesse was, of course, one of the most profound experiences of my life. I know Jesse knew we were there. I did not fully understand what greater purpose was being served but have always felt blessed for the time my wife and I had with him. I've always felt that we are spiritually bonded—he carries a part of me with him and vice versa. He's always been part of the family. Every year, my mother puts his picture on an ornament and hangs it on her Christmas tree with pictures of her other grandchildren.

Our other three children knew at a very early age about their older brother and had to grapple with the concept of death and life after death earlier than most children do. When my second daughter had a medical condition at birth that had a statistically high mortality rate, I called on family in the hereafter, Jesse and my father, to help.

The tenth year after Jesse's passing was a very rough year for my wife. A cousin passed away after a long illness, and her only sibling, a sister, failed to show up for the funeral. We found out later her sister had spent the day going from doctor to doctor, ending up with a diagnosis of leukemia. Soon after, Margaret's father died unexpectedly, and then her sister passed away due to complications following a bone marrow transplant. Margaret and her mother, Grace, were having a hard time dealing with all of this tragedy in such a short period of time.

Five months later, my sister-in-law, Eleanor, who lived in another state, attended a workshop that included an internationally known psychic medium, George Anderson. She learned about the conference because I had given her a subscription to the A.R.E. magazine (the Association for Research and Enlightenment in Virginia Beach, Virginia). Her trip was arranged at the last minute, and I had no clue she was going to attend.

When Mr. Anderson finished his lecture on Saturday morning and started the discernments, baby Jesse was the first soul to speak. Eleanor, as you can imagine, was very surprised to be called up to the front of the room. She almost did not realize the summons was for her. Much of Jesse's communication effort was therefore necessarily focused on explaining his connection to Eleanor. Jesse may have wanted to communicate with my wife and me, but any information he gave that Eleanor could not verify would likely get lost or misinterpreted. In essence, Jesse was restricted to information that Eleanor knew. Also, with hundreds of people in the audience, there was only so much time that could be allotted to one person.

During the discernment, Jesse told Mr. Anderson to give Eleanor a small picture of two children walking across a rickety old wooden bridge while being followed by a large, beautiful angel. Jesse said the picture was to remind us that he is around his sisters like a guardian angel. Eleanor, of course, promptly mailed the painting to us, and we hung it in the girls' bedroom.

Mr. Anderson had brought the picture with him to the conference. While packing his bags for the trip, he had gotten a psychic message to take the picture with him, although he hadn't known why. He realized only during the discernment that it was meant for Eleanor.

Eleanor had attended Jesse's funeral but was not around for the earlier roller coaster ride. She knew some general information but no details. For example, she did not know that Jesse lived for sixteen days (and she could not be expected to know). As a result, a reference to sixteen as Jesse's age was cut off as an avenue of discussion during the discernment because both the psychic and Eleanor assumed that it was a reference to years and did not think about days. In fact, it would appear to most people that the reference was a guess by the psychic that didn't pan out. For us, it was a verification of the authenticity of the communication.

Eleanor's sister, Caitlin, was also at the group workshop when Jesse came through. A year after we lost Jesse, Caitlin had a similar experience with her daughter, Sarah. She had hoped to hear from Sarah at the workshop. Because of our common experience, we had stayed in touch with Caitlin over the years.

Ten months later, my wife, her mother Grace, and I had a private appointment with George Anderson. He was not aware that we had received an earlier message from him about our son.

Here is an excerpt from that taped discernment for Daniel and his family. The initials GA identify Mr. Anderson. Daniel, his wife Margaret, and her mother Grace are identified by the letter D, meaning Daniel, Margaret, Grace, or all three answered the psychic's questions.

One of the ground rules set by Mr. Anderson is that the guests were not to answer his questions with any response other than yes or no, in order to keep the focus on the communications from the other side.

GA: The baby passes in his sleep? Did he go into a coma or sleeplike state? He says he goes into unconsciousness.
D: Yes.
GA: But he had health trouble? Because he says he knew that he was

going to pass on. He says that he had health trouble and goes off into his sleep. He keeps saying, "You couldn't save me." Does that make sense?

D: Yes, I understand.

GA: He says it's not your fault he passed on. He fulfilled and moved on. And you both, as his parents, were part of that fulfillment. Never feel that you failed as parents or anything. You were part of the fulfillment, also.

D: Yes.

GA: You have dreamed about him, yes?

D: I have.

GA: Yes, he says that he has come in dreams. He also says thanks for the memorial and the planting. They're two separate things. There's the memorial or good thing that was done in his memory, and then I saw the book, *A Tree Grows in Brooklyn*. So either a tree has been planted or something has taken root—not necessarily in Brooklyn; that's just my clue. But he says it's the planting as well. He says that he's around your children like a guardian angel.

D: Yes.

GA: Also, there is Sarah?

D: Yes.

GA: Passed on, too?

D: Yes.

GA: Knows both of you. Makes sense?

D: Yes.

GA [to Daniel]: Now wait; she's your family?

D: Yes, sort of.

GA: She keeps coming in as family. She says she knows everybody, but she might mean from over there. So we'll let it go. But she's family by blood?

D: No. [Sarah is the lost baby of Eleanor's sister Caitlin.]

GA: Your little boy had heart trouble? Because he's saying his heart was affected. I feel a lurching at the heart. So he was born with it?

D: Yes.

GA: He said it was there from the start; so I take it must mean he's born with it. Now he shows me the number five. Is he less than five when he passes?

D: Yes.

GA: Yeah, he must have been a baby then or very young. He had trouble breathing?

D: Yes.

GA: I keep getting this heaviness in my chest, which is probably why my heart feels sluggish because it's not getting enough oxygen where it's necessary. Because he even tells me he's not getting enough oxygen to the heart and the brain; so his lungs are doing overtime. He tells me it creates pressure in the head. He says he's seeing fine. Were his eyes affected? Because it's like there's pressure around the eyes. He's saying he's seeing fine now, and then I felt pressure behind the eyes like I had blurred vision even though I can see. But his head was affected; that seems to be the root of the problem. He's not getting enough oxygen, not enough signals to the brain. So apparently, he tells me, the brain and the body aren't working in harmony. I guess he's trying to explain it in the best terms he can. He was on support?

D: Yes.

GA: Because he's like breathing on support, and this is why I think he's in a coma, like here and there. Like in and out of consciousness. He wants to let you know you had no choice but to let him go. "Because you couldn't save me," he says. "There's nothing that could be done." So again, it's not your fault he passed on. Because he was born with this and just seems to become progressively worse, and you're doing everything; so he says don't feel that you've failed as parents. There's nothing you could do.

D: Yes.

GA: Brian? It's funny; your son was talking about a friend, Brian. I think he means over there.

D: Yes?

GA: Your son says he has a common first name. Also Jay? Why is your son showing me the letter J? Does that make sense?

D: Yes.

GA: Oh, he means the letter J, not the name Jay. Am I correct in assuming his first name begins with a J?

D: Yes.

GA: His name is in the Bible?

D: Yes.

GA: He's saying go to the beginning, and I'm asking him Old or New Testament. Again he tells me the name is in the Bible, is that correct?

D: That's correct.

GA: Wait, two of the same letters in the name?

D: Yes.

GA: He says his name is a famous cowboy. [Laughter.] Jesse, from the "roots of Jesse" in the Bible.

D: Yes.

GA: Oh, Jesse James!

D: Yes.

GA: Jes—that's why he's saying you can lower it. He's Jes and Jesse. He keeps coming as baby Jesse. You've heard from him before?

D: Yes.

GA: You know what this means?

D: Yes.

GA: "This is not the first time you've heard from me," he's saying. You've heard from "baby Jesse" before, and he says he addressed himself as such because he tells me—[Mr. Anderson stops in midsentence and asks Daniel and Margaret]—you've never been here before? I wouldn't know, anyway. All right, I'll leave it alone. He says he came before as baby Jesse.

D: Yes.

GA: It's funny; he says, "You've heard my name before." I'll just accept it that I have sometime.

D: Yes.

GA: Now why does Jesse bring up a sister? Does he have one?

D: Yes.

GA: Sisters. Correct? So you have another son?

D: Yes.

GA: You have one son and two daughters.

D: Yes.

GA: He calls out to his sisters and brother, and he comes to them as a guardian angel.

D: Yes.

GA: Your lives are pretty normal, aren't they?

D: Yes.

GA: Except for your son's passing, your lives have certainly been blessed. And as he said, better to have had him for the short time you did than never at all. So, even though you'd rather have him back, it's still a blessing because even for the short time here, he left a big impression. It seems he knew exactly what he was supposed to do, and he fulfilled it only as a baby. [Pause.] I don't understand. He thanks the woman for bringing the message to you.

D: Yes, we understand.

GA: He says he blesses her for bringing the message and a sign from him. That happened last year. Okay, he says he wanted to get it through at a time when you needed to hear that he was all right and at peace. So although he passes as a baby, he's still very spiritual. He comes to me as older because he brings in spiritual wisdom where he seems older than he was here on the Earth.

GA [to Margaret]: You're employed?

D: Yes.

GA: Sometimes you do suffer in silence over him passing to where if you had too much time on your hands, you would have too much time to think about it? Because as Jesse says, one of these days, you're all going to pass on, and he'll see you again someday, just like everybody else. So it's just as he said—like they live in another country, but the only difference is they're not an ocean away; they're closer to all of you than you can ever imagine. Why does he keep holding up a picture of a guardian angel?

D: Yes, we know that.

GA: Because that's his sign that he's around his family like a guardian angel.

D: Yes.

GA: He says something yet again about a guardian angel picture that you have and that you hang it up in remembrance of him.

D: Yes.

GA: Again, he says he came at a time when you needed to hear from him. Just to give you that affirmative shot in the arm, because again, with the exception of him passing, your lives otherwise are pretty normal, yes?

D: Yes.

GA: I mean as much as they can be. It certainly is a difficult burden to carry, but as long as you know he's all right and at peace and in a happy, safe place, it's going to make it easier. You lost a sister [directed to Margaret], yes?

D: Yes.

GA: Your sister's claiming she's like Jesse's mom over there, a motherly figure to him in the hereafter. So she says you don't have to worry about him because your loss is her gain. It's like he lives with her over there. And your daughter [to Grace] keeps calling out to you in love, as a bereaved mother, that she's all right and happy because you do pray for her in your own way, which she thanks you for. She also wishes you happy birthday. Does that make sense?

D: Yes.

GA: Because your daughter does bless you for being so good to her prior to her passing, taking care of her. She also says, "You couldn't save me." Does that make sense? She passes from health troubles. You did everything to save her. She doesn't want you to feel you failed her in any way. You certainly were a good mother, and you definitely helped her. And she and her dad are together in the hereafter. Your daughter says she's back to her old self. She says she passes in her sleep? You do pray for her in your own way, which she does thank you for. Kaddish has been said for her? [Kaddish is an ancient Jewish prayer said for loved ones for the first eleven months following their passing.] She says [to Grace], "Thank you for the mitzvah [a good deed] in my name, because you and she were close; you were not only mother and daughter, but you were great pals." Also [to Daniel and Margaret], was there another loss of a son?

D: Yes.

GA: Wait a minute, somebody just walked in the room and said, "I'm the son that passed on." Is that correct? Did you have a miscarriage or something like that?

D: Yeah.

GA: You lost more than one child? Before birth, though? Because this one comes in before birth. I think had the cycle of birth continued, you would have had a son. It could be miscarriage, abortion, whatever. The soul is in the room claiming to be Jesse's brother. It would have been the soul that would have entered the body had the cycle of birth continued. Apparently, he is there as well; makes sense? But Jesse embraces the three of you with love and his sisters and brother also. They all, all those who've been here, send you great love before they leave.

Daniel continues: Mr. Anderson had said during the group session that Jesse had a friend with him named Brian, who said hello. We had no clue who that could be. As my wife and I were talking, trying to figure out all the names, Eleanor overheard and recognized the name Brian. She informed us that her sister, Shauna, had had a baby named Brian who had passed away shortly after birth several years before Jesse was born.

In addition, Mr. Anderson said, "Someone walked into the room and said, 'I'm the son that passed on.' This one comes in as passing on before birth. If he had gone to full term he would have been a boy." He was claiming to be the brother of Jesse. "Have you had a miscarriage?" Mr. Anderson asked.

We weren't expecting to hear from the miscarried baby, and so it took us by surprise. Margaret had had a miscarriage. We were delighted that he came to say hello. We named our miscarried baby Samuel the next morning. Perhaps, had our session gone longer, we would have heard more. I know that my son's efforts to contact us were not only acts of love but service to God. Statements he made in the second session confirm that he was clearly aware of the benefits that his communication would bring. In sharing this with others, I'm just following my cue to carry through with the work God started through Jesse.

All things have a purpose, even a sixteen-day life or a miscarriage. I trust you have heard from many others. It is not as isolated an occurrence as most people may think.

From the correspondence I've received, it certainly seems that communication experiences are more common than some might think. Phaedra, who shared an earlier story of a dream of her baby girl, also wrote about seeing her friend's baby, Jeremiah, during a psychometry reading. A psychic reader using psychometry has the ability to sense thoughts, feelings, or images by holding a personal possession belonging to the subject of the reading.

Phaedra and Friend's Baby Jeremiah

I am able to do psychometry, although I do resist unless someone practically begs me. My son's friend asked me to do her ring, and I saw the most beautiful baby fairy, all dressed in green. I told her that I had never seen a fairy before and it was quite a novel experience for me. He said (in thought transference) that his name was Jeremiah, and I related that to her.

She asked what he looked like, and I told her he had dark hair and eyes and was a very beautiful, chubby baby. She started crying and said she had had a baby boy named Jeremiah who had died, a crib death. I had not known that and felt bad for bringing news that made her so sad. The baby sent me a thought to tell her that he was happy where he was.

In Tracey's story, the baby girl herself seems to be the psychic.

Tracey and Baby Girl

In December 1966, after having carried a baby girl for six months, I went into pre-term labor, and my daughter lived for less than an hour.

About eight years later, I was talking with my roommate about pregnancies and due dates, and she mentioned that her daughter, with whom I'd become very close, had been due on the ides of March in 1967. When she told me that, I told her that it seemed an amazing coincidence that my daughter had been due the same day and year. Her daughter had walked into the room during our discussion and casually said, "That was me! That was the only way I could have you both for my mother—you each carried me for part of the time."

Kelly wrote that her baby Avery came through in a psychic reading to tell her she was being taken care of and that she would be returning to her. Additionally, Kelly's young daughter tells her of seeing the baby frequently.

Kelly and Baby Avery

I lost my baby in October 2002, when I was twelve weeks pregnant. About six months later, my mother and sister went to see a psychic. The man told them that a baby had died in our family and that it was okay because her great-grandmother was taking care of her now. (My grandmother had died several years earlier, and she was the one talking to the psychic.) He also said that when I get pregnant again, it will be with twins: my baby and my grandmother coming back to me.

Then about two days ago, my two-year-old daughter, Sallie, and I were playing. I wrote the name Avery, which we named our angel, on her leg. She said out of the blue, "Mommy, Avery is at the door." I asked, "Do you see Avery, Sallie?" and she said in a matter-of-fact way, "Yeah, Mommy, all the time." I told my mother, and the next day she asked Sallie whether Avery was a boy or a girl, and Sallie replied, "A girl, silly."

Messages in Visions

Some mothers have seen visions of their unborn children. Chris related this story, as told to her by her aunt, about an experience her now-deceased grandmother had with a baby girl she lost.

Chris and Grandmother's Baby Girl

This story is my grandmother's, and if she could, she'd be writing it. She passed in 1977. Sometime after my aunt was born in 1931 and before my mother was born in 1947, my grandmother miscarried a baby girl.

The way my aunt told me this tale is, my grandmother had always been an early riser. She would get up before everyone else to enjoy a cup of coffee, sitting quietly, before cooking breakfast. One morning, as she looked out the kitchen window, she saw a little girl swinging on the swing set. Upon seeing my grandmother in the window, the girl's halo became evident. She was dressed in white lace and had long, dark, curly hair. She swung a little longer, raised her hand to say good-bye, and disappeared. My grandmother knew at that moment she was going to lose the child she was carrying and that it was a girl. That same afternoon, she miscarried.

I don't know how my grandmother felt at that moment, but I would have been glad that the little girl had said good-bye.

Cina shares her story of the painful loss of her son Michael. Nearly twenty years later, he appeared to her during a difficult time to reassure her that everything would be all right.

Cina and Baby Michael

Very few people know about this incident with my former husband, but I owe it to my son to tell the truth. In 1979, I moved to Texas with my husband and two girls. We had been living there for about four months when I found out I was pregnant. I was overjoyed with the news. I was married very young to my high school sweetheart and wanted nothing more than to have a boy. I was never told that my baby was a boy, but somehow I knew that he was.

My husband did not want another child. One day, he came home from work and invited me to go to a place called Dinosaur Mountain. We left the girls with his brother, who was visiting us at the time. I went with him, since it was a serene place where a stream ran through the valley. When we arrived, he took me by the hand and pulled me up the mountain and down again, against my will. When we returned home, I went into labor, and he refused to take me to the hospital. Keep in mind I was twenty-three years old. I had my son while I was lying on my bed. When he was delivered, my husband took my son outside and buried him. I knew it was a boy. I was approximately three to four months pregnant at the time.

I can't remember too much about the three days after that. I was on the verge of a nervous breakdown. I would sit on my bed and cry uncontrollably. After about the third day, I was on the bed crying and heard a knock on my closet door. I didn't look up and kept crying. Then I heard three more very loud knocks. A calming spirit moved over me, and after that, I began to get some control of myself. I don't know what the knocking was, but it had a major calming effect on me. I moved back home to North Carolina, separating from my husband.

In 1986, I remarried, and we opened a business. In 1998, the business went bankrupt, and my husband and I separated. Again, I was alone and at my wits' end. I went to bed one night and prayed for God to let me die. For some reason, during this entire ordeal, my son was on my mind. I was not asleep during my son's visit. My son walked up to my bed, touched the side of my face, and said, "It will be okay, Mamma." It was for a brief moment, but no one will ever know what those few seconds meant to me.

He presented to me at the age he would have been had he been living, not as a child, which was astonishing to me since I had always felt that if I ever saw him, he would still be a baby. He was a handsome young man, and very gentle. His features were similar to those of one of my cousins. I would give anything to see him again, but that brief moment was more than I could have ever asked for. I now have a grandson (the only boy in the family), and I look at him and wonder whether my son would have looked like my grandson as a child. I never spent a living moment with my son, but I love and miss him as though I had spent my life with him. He will always be in my heart and mind, and I look forward to seeing him again one day.

It took me two years before I could talk about this, even to my mother. My soul yearns for him, but I know he is in a wonderful place.

In the next story, Natalie's four-year-old daughter tells her she talks to her "friend" in the mirror, a little boy named Darien.

Natalie and Baby Darien

I never thought I would be writing such a letter because I thought no one else would believe me. I myself have not heard from my son Darien, who was stillborn ten years ago, but my nearly five-year-old daughter has. She has been talking into a mirror to her "friend," and we thought it was just her imagination, until one day she woke up in the middle of the night and said the little boy kept talking to her and telling her that something bad was going to happen.

Two days later, my great-uncle died. When we asked my daughter the little boy's name, she said it was Darien. We had never told her his name before.

MESSAGES THROUGH MEDITATION

Meditation raises our conscious awareness in many aspects of our lives. It is defined as deep contemplation or reflection, introspection, or pondering. In spiritual meditation, one clears the mind and remains still and silent for a period of time, seeking to attain a higher level of consciousness or connection with a higher power. Meditation can also bring about an altered state, enabling communication with the other side. Many methods and goals of meditation exist, almost as many as there are believers in its power.

Stacey tells her story of finding closure through hearing from her baby girl Colestine during meditation.

Stacey and Baby Colestine

I found out at five and a half weeks into my pregnancy that my HCG levels were dropping and I would miscarry my baby. I waited for days for the baby to pass, but nothing happened.

I went to see a very dear friend who is a Reiki master and meditation guide. [Reiki is healing technique based on the principle that the therapist can channel energy into the patient by means of touch, to activate the natural healing processes of the patient's body.] I don't know what I expected, but I was not expecting to hear from the baby. I just needed to find peace at that moment and was anxious to feel better. I had just had a Reiki session before the meditation.

During the meditation, I got an image of a crystal clear fallopian tube.

Actually, it resembled a crystal ornament rather than a human organ, but that is how meditations are. I worried about an ectopic pregnancy.

At the very end of our meditation, a very clear voice said to me, "Good-bye, Mommy; good-bye." It was a girl's voice, and it was so clear and loud. Waves of emotion came over me when I heard the sweet voice. I have no doubt it was my little girl. When I did come out of the meditation, I was crying, and so was my guide. It was a beautiful moment. That night, I started to pass the baby. Within a couple of days, the dear one was gone.

I had been given some insight into my child-to-be in previous meditations and had actually seen her. I was told her name was Colestine. So I have always thought of this lost child as being Colestine.

I shared this story with my guide and with my husband, and other than them, only you. I don't know that most people could appreciate or believe this story.

A Reiki master from South America, Maria, wrote to me about her meditation experiences of seeing her baby girl Leonor, whom she had lost thirty-three years earlier.

Maria and Baby Leonor

In 1966, my fiancé and I decided to get married the following summer. We were going to wait to start a family, and so I made an appointment with a doctor to go on birth control pills. After the exam, I got up from the table bleeding. I had never had such an exam, and I didn't know what had happened.

We decided that I should not go on the pill after all, more his will than mine, and I got pregnant again. I say again because this time I realized that I had been pregnant before and had lost the baby when I'd had the examination and bled profusely. This time I knew from the beginning because I started feeling something similar to what I had felt before my doctor visit asking for birth control.

Time passed, and I began meditating. In meditation, I saw a little girl. She was with my deceased mother, and I thought at first she was me as a little girl because she looked a little like me when I was five or six years old, but she was more beautiful. Then I realized it was the baby girl

I'd lost, the baby girl I'd always wanted. She said thanks for giving her the opportunity to live at the time she needed to. Her unspoken message was love.

Another time in meditation, she was with my brother, who had passed away many years ago. He and I had always been very close. Sometimes I even feel her kissing or embracing me. Yesterday I saw her with my eyes open!

As I write to you, I can feel her by my side, telling me she is closer to me this way because there is no time or space limiting our connection. Her love is constant and unconditional.

I felt guilt for a long time, not knowing I was pregnant and going to the doctor and losing her on the table, but I feel different now. I now know I had nothing to do with it, but you know how we tend to punish ourselves.

I know in my heart that when our loved ones go on to the next dimension, they are even closer to us than in this one. We can communicate with them more easily and profoundly.

It means a lot to me to talk with you about this subject. I don't usually share my experiences with anybody outside of my closest friends—and sometimes not even with them. But I felt it was time to tell you because you are reaching out to mothers who are deeply hurt over the loss of a child. Now they will know their children are still so close to them. All they have to do is open their hearts, and they will feel this warm and tender love that is waiting for acknowledgment.

Please write the book and tell the mothers the beauty of the spiritual life. Not many people understand or believe the reality of it, but still we must pass on the message, and whoever has ears will hear.

Annette had miscarried three months prior to reading about my research. She wrote about her experience of communicating with her baby as she breathed with her contractions. Focused deep breathing can bring about an altered state.

Annette and Baby

I felt as though something wasn't right with my pregnancy of about six or seven weeks, and therefore I wasn't surprised—though I was sad and disappointed—when I started spotting. I went home and lay down, with my two-year-old daughter nursing herself to sleep. I had done Bradley classes [a method of natural childbirth without the use of drugs] before my daughter was born and used some of these techniques. I got in touch with my body and said a little prayer. I told God that I would accept whatever was meant to be and asked for the strength to deal with whatever that was. I spoke with my body and told it that I knew it had the wisdom to do what it needed to do.

Shortly afterwards, I felt some contractions, which I breathed with. I knew when I had passed the baby, and I felt the presence of that spirit. I communicated to the baby, "I am sorry that this was not the right time or the right body for you. I hope you will join us again soon. I love you." In return, I was completely filled with the most wonderful feeling of peace and love. I felt the baby communicate to me that everything was as it was meant to be. That feeling of peace and love was so strong that I felt blessed by the whole experience and was able to accept it easily.

Before becoming pregnant with my daughter, I'd had a miscarriage that was extremely upsetting for me, but this time, I felt so fortunate. The communication with the spirit of the baby was so strong and fulfilling that I feel calm and peaceful whenever I think of it.

Born and raised in the Philippines, Nellie came to the United States in 1992. She holds a master's degree in economics and speaks five languages. Here is her story of her baby boy.

Nellie and Baby Boy

I had an encounter with my unborn child last year. First, I have to tell you that I am new to this spirit stuff. October of 2000 is when I finally was able to meditate for the first time. I'd tried for years but couldn't do it.

I got pregnant in December 2001. Since I don't work, I had more time for meditation. One day when I was less than three months pregnant, while my eyes were closed but I wasn't asleep, I saw my baby's silhouette. It was moving as if it were swimming. I got scared and opened my eyes.

Then one afternoon when I was more than three months pregnant, I lay down on the couch in the living room for my afternoon meditation. I fell asleep, probably for fifteen minutes. I know I didn't sleep more than that, since I was awakened by the clicking sound of my guided meditation tape. I opened my eyes and decided to close them again, attempting to continue my nap. When I closed my eyes, I saw my baby smiling. This time he had a distinct face. A bright yellow background surrounded him, and outside of that background was a bright dark blue background. I was terrified but didn't attempt to open my eyes. I was enjoying it. Then I wanted to make sure I wasn't dreaming, and so I opened my eyes. I can't describe the feeling. It was a mixture of being thrilled and scared. I closed my eyes again and saw the same thing. It just wouldn't go away. I was pretty sure the baby was a boy. (I'd had that feeling the day I found out I was pregnant.) I opened my eyes again and looked around the living room to see whether there was a bright yellow or dark blue color, but there wasn't. So I closed my eyes again, and as expected, I saw my baby again. Then, after a while, the baby disappeared. One thing I was very sure about that day was that I knew I wasn't dreaming. Less than three weeks after that incident, my baby died inside me, and yes, I was right: he was a baby boy. To this day I still don't understand why my baby appeared to me and died after a few weeks. Was he trying to tell me that he wouldn't be able to stay long? I don't know.

A few days after my miscarriage, I saw him again in a dream, walking with my father, who died in 1992. They were walking by a lake or some kind of body of water.

Messages through Near–Death Experiences

As described in several published books, near-death experiences have occurred in individuals who were clinically dead but were revived, as well as in those who believed they were about to die but survived. On regaining consciousness, these people tell of feeling deep peace and unconditional love, as well as meeting departed loved ones and seeing visions of an afterlife, often while being in extraordinarily bright light.

One of the earliest researchers into near-death experiences is Raymond Moody, MD. In his book *Life After Life*, he reports on his investigation of more than one hundred cases of persons who were clinically dead and later revived.

Karen wrote to me about her little girl Jessica who had a near-death experience at five years old during which she saw her miscarried brother. Her mother Karen tells Jessica's story of baby James.

Karen, Jessica and Baby James

I have two beautiful children, Jessica and Frank. Before Jessica was born, she had a brother, James, who was born at twenty-four weeks and died instantly when he was delivered.

One day, my husband, also named Frank, and Jessica, then five, were in the pool. Frank turned around for a minute, and when he looked back Jessica was under the water motionless. Frank saved her by doing CPR.

A week after the accident, Jessica told me that James told her to stay here and take care of Frank and me. She asked me whether she had a brother James, and I said, "Yes, he's an angel in heaven."

Frank and I had never told her about her brother because it was just a sad chapter in our lives. When Jessica started talking about him, how God took him for a special reason, I was just amazed. She explained that wherever she went, no harm would come to her, and it hasn't. Jessica sends James kisses before she goes to bed because she knows he saved her that day, and I am forever grateful to him. He is missed, but I know he is here watching me.

Messages Through Hypnosis

Ihad become a certified hypnotist and had been practicing for three years when I met Jennifer, who is an artist. On her way home from work one day, Jennifer felt drawn to pull over to a small local bookstore. Once there, she immediately saw my hypnosis brochure.

She set up an appointment and came to my office, saying she wanted to establish contact with a daughter she lost due to crib death eighteen years earlier, because she wanted to move on with her life. Jennifer added that one month prior to the baby's death, she dreamed the baby would die. After the baby died, she came to Jennifer in her dreams.

While hypnotized, Jennifer saw and spoke to her daughter, Monica, in her inner mind. In her hypnotized state, Jennifer told me what she'd learned.

Jennifer and Baby Monica

She's beautiful. She has my face, long hair, so pretty; she's tall. She's in a white gown. She's right here. She's holding my face. She's so pretty. She didn't want to be here. She wanted to go home. She's with me all the time. She told me she was only going to be here for a while. She tried to prepare me. She's holding me. [Long pause.] Oh, angels! I'm so loved. [Long pause.] It wasn't my fault. She wanted me to know what true love was. She's here for me because I have a special heart. My journey is going to be hard, or was hard in the past. She's never going to leave me.

She wanted to come be with me. She told me not to grieve for her anymore, that she'll always be here. Paint her picture. She'll help me.

The angels are touching me—you can feel such love. She said I'll always be her mommy. Funny, I feel like the little child. There's such a white light. Oh, they're all going. [I have goose bumps as she says this.] She's kissing my cheek. She sends messages—to listen to my inner heart.

We're the same height. She parts her hair on the side. She has high cheekbones, a pointy chin. [Long pause.] They've all been lessons.

She says I should be free. Her leaving wasn't my decision; it was hers. She's re-walking the hospital room. A long hallway. The hallway was her way to heaven, and I walked her halfway there. She tells me the tears are good. They cleanse the soul. When I'm crying, she's there. I'm not alone. She's hugging me. She's going.

Several months later, Jennifer's co-worker told me that Jennifer felt healed as a result of her session with me.

Sunny and Sister's Baby Carmen

As though some kind of invisible invitation had been sent, more mothers of lost babies were apparently finding their way to me. Over my years of practice, I had studied every book I could find on past-life regressions, especially those of Dr. Brian Weiss, author of *Many Lives, Many Masters*. In addition, I had received hundreds of hours of professional training in regression by some of the best people in the country, including Dr. Weiss. And although I had several years of experience guiding others into past lives, often with clients speaking to their guides, nothing in my background fully prepared me for what was about to happen when Sunny walked into my office.

Astounding messages from a friend named Eli emerged during the appointment Sunny had set up with me for smoking cessation. And somehow, a healing for Sunny's sister, especially for the loss of her baby Carmen, resulted from our session. I had guided Sunny into a hypnotic state, and we did the work for her to stop smoking, but just as I was about to begin my next sentence to emerge her, she said, "I'm in space, surrounded by stars and planets. I see a door."

It took me by surprise. I often use doors to go into other lifetimes, but she had no way of knowing that. Something was happening, and I was curious to find out what it was.

"Sunny, is there something behind the door that will assist you to stop smoking?" I inquired.

"I don't know. I just feel pulled to it," she replied.

"Open the door and walk in. Tell me what you see," I asked.

"Ah, green." She breathed out the words as she exhaled. "Birds are singing. I'm home." Tears began rolling down her cheeks as a blissful look came over her face.

"Become aware of your feet and notice what, if anything, you are wearing on them," I instructed.

"Sandals."

"Are your feet big or small?"

"Small."

"How old are you?" I asked.

"Twelve," she replied. "I'm at a well. There are women there. I was taken, but I've come to tell my mother I'm fine. She sees me."

Questions raced through my mind. It seemed she had spontaneously regressed to a different time period. Some view this kind of experience as a metaphor or psychodrama of the mind, while others who believe in reincarnation see it as a past life.

Questions raced through my mind. Was it Sunny? How did she find her way back home after being taken? What country did she live in? As though she had heard the questions in my mind, she answered.

"My name is Marishá," she told me. "Oh," she interjected, sounding surprised, "my mother is Rhonda [her sister in this life]. She has ancient fear and worry." [It wasn't until I emerged her from hypnosis that I learned her sister suffered from anxieties.] "Oh, my friend is here," she related, seemingly elated. "He says that as a result of the work we did, my sister will heal. He wants to speak. His name is Eli, and I told him it was okay to speak."

Her face contorted slightly as her voice lowered, and she became more serious. I held my pen steady to my notepad as I waited for Eli to speak.

"This is a time of great turmoil on your planet." Eli began. "Be sure that this is a transition to a higher phase of humanity. We are helping you develop to the next level. Your highest good is in mind. Your guides are near. It won't be long before peace, serenity, and knowledge are finally achieved by your race. In trust and love you will achieve a new level of humanity that transcends countries, peoples, and planets. We are all truly one."

The terrorist attack of 9/11 had occurred only two weeks prior, and I sensed his words referred to it. During my initial interview with Sunny, we had discussed that she was not involved in the churches of her childhood, but nothing she said gave me any indication she'd be capable of the depth of Eli's words. His next words made the hair on my neck stand on end.

"Take my blessing, Patricia. You are on the correct path. Walk boldly forward. Put your fears aside. We will be guiding you."

I immediately knew the message had to do with writing the book. I emerged Sunny, and she opened her eyes. "Wow!" [Long pause.] "Do you understand his message to you?" she asked.

"Yes, I do," I answered solemnly, without elaborating, and asked whether she was aware of what had just happened.

"Yes, it was as though I was hearing him talk to you as a third party," she replied.

Knowing she received more information than she shared with me during the regression, I asked, "Help me understand what happened to Marishá. How did she escape?"

"I didn't escape," she explained. "I came back in spirit form to tell my mother I was fine so she wouldn't worry. She saw my spirit at the well."

We talked about Eli's message as I tried to comprehend the magnitude of what had just happened. Had her guide actually talked to me directly? I knew such revelations could happen, of course. I just didn't think they would happen to me.

Several months later, Sunny called for an appointment to help motivate her to exercise. She also told me that a lot had happened since our last session, and she was excited that she no longer smoked, but she had more important information to tell me.

Sunny had spoken to her sister, who told her that the day before had been the anniversary of the death of her baby, Carmen, stillborn at seven and a half months, a loss she'd mourned for fourteen years. But what was different that morning was that she wasn't sad. It was the first time she hadn't cried her eyes out on the baby's anniversary. She'd gone to Carmen's grave as she had all those years but hadn't cried. Although perplexed by her lack of pain, she spoke to baby Carmen and, for the first time, knew she was okay.

Excitedly, she'd also told Sunny that all her anxieties were gone. Even more amazing to Sunny was that her sister was open to hearing about Sunny's past-life regression experience, information that would have made her uncomfortable in the past.

When Sunny mentioned the reason for her sister's anxiety problem—the loss of the baby—I knew why she had found her way to my office. I was stunned but happy for the healing that had occurred for her sister, a healing that Eli said would happen. In fact, baby Carmen has come to Sunny's sister often, and they now have a relationship. Carmen has even offered to help a sibling who is having problems.

"Eli has come to me several times since our session," Sunny reported. Eli had told her that I have a companion, a best friend, something with an L. "She is with you every second and is a great help with your book. Let her be an active help. She has golden honey hair and sparkling eyes, and she just adores you."

I asked Sunny about her religious background and beliefs. "I was a Fundamentalist Pentecostal Christian," she began. "I now view it as a time when I got scared, when I wanted to feel safe. I began doing missionary work with the church and started seeing other people's pain. I had a rigid code based on the Ten Commandments and chose to close myself in a box. After my failure to be the perfect Christian I was expected to be, I was so disappointed in myself that my paradigm shifted. That was five years ago. I stopped going to church, and then several years later, I went to school and studied world religions, discovering there was a thread of truth in all of them. I no longer believe in hell. I believe demons are made when we manifest them. We get what we expect. We're made of the same stuff as God."

As fascinated as I was with our conversation, I knew we had to begin to work on the reason she had come back to see me, which was to motivate her to exercise. I did a rapid induction with her, and she immediately began beaming. "Eli's here," she whispered. I swallowed hard. Eli briefly mentioned my book, but then another entity started to speak.

"I'm Leeann," she began. I was surprised it wasn't Eli but delighted to learn about Leeann. "I'm appointed to be your companion," she told me. "We've been down many roads. It's my turn to be your helper. I know how badly your heart was broken." [Instinctively I knew she was referring to my loss of Dillon. I felt my throat tighten as hot tears welled in my eyes.] "You can trust that the healing keeps going on." [Pause.] "He's very happy—the boy. His hair goes over his forehead. He's nine or ten." [This was the age Dillon would have been had he lived.] "You've been given a gift to be able to see into the hearts of others. I'll help you develop this gift. We'll have a lot of fun if you're open. I'll help you meet others to help as well, but I'm the first. I can help you with decisions and intuition with helping people. I want you to know I love you very much."

"She's so happy," Sunny said. "The boy is with Leeann."

"What's his name?" I asked slowly.

"Ryan," she answered. [Strange, that was the name I had wanted for the baby.] "He feels very fulfilled. He's a laughing boy."

Unable to resist, I had to ask, "Does he go by another name?"

"Evan," she replied. "He said he has many names. He's laughing as if he knows something I don't."

"Does he go by a name that begins with a D?" I asked, trying to get clarity on who the boy was, but not wanting to lead her.

"Dillon," she immediately responded. I felt the blood rush out of my face. "He's smiling at me," she continued. A single tear ran down my right cheek.

"Tell him I saw the key," I whispered.

"They're not out there—they're a part of you already. All it takes is a moment, a breath, and they're there," Sunny said, referring to the spirits of departed loved ones.

After a long pause, she began again, "Leeann is planning to introduce you to some of the children as the mothers are brought to you. They're a lot of Dillon's friends. They're going to have a huge impact on allowing people to understand. When children move beyond this place, they don't miss us or grieve for us. They feel only great comfort and joy because we understand. They are aware of us, concerned for us. They feel only deep joy and trust in the creator. Every time a child leaves this place, it's because he chose to before he came. So guilt and shame are useless [meaning for the mother and father]."

"We have agreements with others for our experiences," Sunny continued. "Part of our growth can come only through pain. Some come only briefly so that others can learn from the experience of love, and it's hard for us to accept that we volunteer for such duty. Many times a group of souls will agree and plan, like a team planning the scenarios, but there will always be free will. Every single moment, our creator is encouraging the souls, filling them with strength and energy, and bathing everyone with incredible love."

I emerged Sunny from hypnosis. "I'm doing some writing, Sunny," I told her and asked, "Do you know what it is about?"

"It's about mothers who've lost very little babies," she replied, "even before birth." Sunny had no way of knowing about my miscarriage or the book.

Years passed before I spoke to Sunny again. She told me the reason she hadn't contacted me was because she'd become frightened. Her family looked on her as if she'd lost her mind when she told them what had happened, even though she felt she'd learned what reality was through our sessions.

Now Sunny looked at me solemnly, saying, "You are the key to open the door, the catalyst, the bridge for others to find the spiritual side." In the intervening years, Sunny herself had become psychic and could see and hear the other side.

"Dillon's here," she told me. "He's a dancing, mischievous boy," she added with a chuckle. "He's saying, 'Be sure to tell her I'm so proud of her, and all us kids are glad she's doing it. The book will lift the spirits of those who've lost babies. Death is just a doorway.'" Sunny paused and then added, "They get such joy in helping you," before Dillon spoke again.

"We kids thank you," he said. "You're going to get feedback years from now. You'll help heal the mommies."

His last words jogged my memory of what Maryanne had told me Dillon had said years earlier. I replayed that message silently in my mind. "One of your life's missions is to write a book. The name of the book will be *Angel Babies*, to help heal the mommies who've lost their babies."

As Sunny had related in one of our sessions, guilt and shame are useless for mothers or fathers, yet many mothers carry guilt over the loss of a baby, whether through miscarriage or abortion. Guilt feelings are often released when mothers gain understanding about their babies' leaving, as Cheryl's story illustrates. She relates her experience of talking to her baby while in hypnosis and asking for the baby's forgiveness.

Cheryl and Baby

I am quite open about my personal matters, probably because I have truly healed those issues and no longer feel any shame. I am confident in how I feel, and so I am not afraid to tell people about my experiences. I think it is time for society to be honest about what happens in it. I consider myself very spiritual, and some of my spirituality relates to metaphysical aspects. I believe in reincarnation and that we choose our parents and our parents choose us. Of course, that happens on some other level that we are not consciously aware of in this life. Your research sounds exciting, and I am glad to hear you are taking the time to focus on this issue. I feel many women today carry around a guilt that is unnecessary.

Here is my story. I was attending a hypnosis class where the instructor was explaining how to use chair therapy in the process of forgiving. We had touched on the topic of how we should ask our female clients whether or not they had any pregnancies that did not come to full term due to abortion or miscarriage, in order to deal with any hidden guilt or grief.

He began to describe how to do the chair therapy with them by putting the unborn baby in the chair in front of them. He had explained that in many experiences, the baby was almost always very jovial and happy and given to good-natured teasing. One minute I was taking notes diligently, and the next minute I fell apart in my chair, tears streaming uncontrollably down my face. See, I was always comfortable with the decision that I'd made. My parents did not like my decision to have an abortion but supported me through it all the way. My friends knew and were fine with it as well. My boyfriend at the time was also in agreement. I knew deep in my soul that the time was not right and having the abortion was the right thing to do.

When the procedure was over and I was in the recovery room, every woman was upset and crying except for me. After a while, I began feeling guilty because I had not felt guilty. Somehow, what the instructor said that day moved something deep inside me, and the emotion broke through. I had a personal hypnosis session the next day, and I put my unborn baby in the chair. The baby was more of a presence felt than an actual baby in a chair and was more like a one-year-old than a newborn. I did not get a male/female sense. I would compare the feeling to seeing someone in a dream that you see as a man, but it is not so much what he looks like as the presence that you feel about the person. It's as if you know the person, but you could not describe what he or she looks like because that is not important at the time. It is the essence that comes through, not the physical characteristics. That is what it was like with the baby. I felt it was someone I knew but could not describe.

The baby was laughing and was very happy. It explained that I should not be sorry about anything, that we made the decision together. It was not just my choice but its choice also. It agreed it was not the right time and that it was comfortable just where it was. It said we would meet again when the time was right. The baby made me feel at peace. I went through the forgiveness process, but the baby made me feel there was nothing to forgive, that I had done nothing wrong.

If you ask me whether I spoke to the spirit of the baby, I would have to say, for lack of better understanding, yes, it was like that. I also feel it was possible that I remembered a conversation that occurred on a subconscious level when the decision to have the abortion was made. Either way or both ways, there was definitely a strong connection with that spirit. The spirit was familiar, as if I had known it before. The baby also said it was watching me and protecting me. I do believe that we have soul groups [souls who reincarnate together], and so I would have to assume that spirit is in mine. Needless to say, it was a wonderful experience.

During a training workshop on past-life regression at an international conference, I met Victor Borak, a medical doctor from Argentina. I told him about the book I was working on. Although he thought my experiences were interesting, he later revealed that he thought they were a little strange—until he regressed a female patient to the interlife period [the time between lives or incarnations]. Here's the story he related.

Dr. Victor Borak's Patient

I've been working with a patient, and during one of our sessions, I took her to the interlife, just before this lifetime. She told me at first that she didn't know where she was, but then she told me she was in the uterus. When I asked her whether it was her mother's, she suddenly began to cry, saying, "No, I'm in another uterus, but I didn't make it. I died before I was born. I had a twin brother who survived, but I didn't." She couldn't stop crying and then said, "When I went to the light, I learned that the episode would be of great importance to the mother and brother."

Dr. Brian Weiss' Workshop

At another conference, I attended a past-life regression workshop with Dr. Brian Weiss, who wanted us to understand that we all have psychic ability. He wanted to illustrate his point through the use of psychometry. We were to find a partner, ideally someone we didn't know, and exchange a piece of jewelry. While we were holding the items, he guided us into hypnosis, telling us to notice everything we saw, felt, or heard, no matter how strange. Afterwards, we were to talk about all those images or feelings with our partner. He stressed that we should share everything with our partner and not hold back any information we received, since even the smallest thing could be important. I had practiced pyschometry only once before in a similar situation and had been surprised by my accuracy. So I looked forward to another experience, curious whether I'd be accurate again.

Holding my partner's bracelet, I allowed myself to be guided into hypnosis. I immediately saw a scene. I was looking at a field of long, golden grass. In the distance was a forest of sorts. A huge tree with wide limbs stood in the forefront of the field, slightly to the left. I assumed it was a place in northern Florida where the woman lived, because the tree was larger than most seen along Florida's coastline, and I found myself admiring the site. I wondered whether this place was special to my partner and thought I should notice everything so I could describe it to her in detail. I glanced to the right and noticed the trees in the far distance before looking back to the big tree, where I saw a baby.

I thought the woman would want to know the sex of the child, and I wondered whether she was a mother-to-be. First I saw a baby boy and then a baby girl. *Which is it?* I wondered. Both babies appeared again, and I was frustrated I didn't have a definitive answer, thinking I had to choose one.

I looked once again to the distant forest to the right and then back to the tree in the forefront. This time a little girl stood under the tree. She appeared to be about three years old and was very happily twirling in circles under the tree. I noted her shoulder-length blonde hair. Again I glanced at the forest and then back to the tree. This time, there was a young girl, about seven years old, standing at the tree. I knew this could not be the same child because her hair was nearly black.

I glanced away and then back to the tree again. Now all the children were together under the tree, and the three-year-old was still gleefully twirling. The dark-haired girl stood looking directly at me as though she could see me looking at her. She was holding a baby and looking intently at me as if to say, "I have the baby." The images were very clear, and I was certain my experience would have meaning for my partner.

When I told her what I saw, she emphatically said none of it made sense to her. I was surprised by her response and a little disappointed. The children didn't look like anyone I knew. Was my ego involved? I couldn't let go of the clear images of the children's faces in my mind, and I was certain I had never seen that scene or the children before. And then a thought popped in my mind. I leaned over and asked, "Have you lost a baby?"

She sighed deeply before replying slowly, "Not exactly *lost* ..." I mouthed the word *abortion*. With that, she began sobbing.

"Were there four?" she asked. I assured her they were all well and that the oldest daughter was holding the baby.

Some people attended the workshop, but of all the people present, she sat next to me. Who else would have thought of the lost babies? There are no coincidences.

Messages through Coincidences

A coincidence is defined as an accidental and remarkable occurrence of events or ideas at the same time, in a way that sometimes suggests a causal relationship. I've also heard it said that coincidences are God's way of remaining anonymous. For me, one thing is certain: something much greater than ourselves is at work when we experience coincidences.

Carla wrote me from Salt Lake City, Utah, describing herself as an atheist who believes in life after life. She told me about her baby Isobella.

Carla and Baby Isobella

I have had three miscarriages in the last year but have only felt the presence of the first baby. I have considered the possibility that the same baby may keep trying to come down. I had contact for about one year and nothing since.

In September 1999, I found out I was pregnant. I wasn't surprised when the test came back positive since I'd been feeling the unmistakable sickness for a week, but I was elated to have it confirmed. I told family and friends the good news. It was amazing how fast the little baby started making changes in my life. I dreamed of holding the baby and wondered whether it was a boy or girl. I determined the due date, and I got the baby clothes out of storage to see what we had and what we'd need.

My teenager, just turning sixteen then, was excited, and so were my husband and friends who knew of my struggles with infertility. They were calling by the day to offer congratulations.

I cherished knowing that there was a baby growing in me. I loved to place my hand on my abdomen and say, "Hi, baby. I love you," though it sounds silly, I know. We'd go to the park on Saturdays, and I'd walk around with my head in the clouds, so happy.

Little did I know that tragedy was already in progress. I didn't feel quite as sick as I had the day before, but I told myself that it was okay to have good days and sick days. I wasn't concerned. We had a birthday party to celebrate our son's sixteen years, and the next day I started spotting. The horror of finding blood is something I'll never forget; the shock made me physically dizzy. I called my husband at work and asked him to bring home a pregnancy test. I thought if it were still positive then maybe the spotting would stop. Implantation bleeding, I told myself. It was positive, and so I went to bed feeling that maybe everything would be okay. The next four days were awful as I waited for the spotting to stop, afraid to visit the bathroom in case the bleeding had become worse. I went from convincing myself that the baby was fine to knowing that it wasn't.

On Friday morning, my worst fear came about: heavy bleeding was the obvious sign that a miscarriage was inevitable. One of the hardest times I've lived through followed. I was surprised at the severity of my emotions. It was difficult to realize there would be no baby in May and that I would never hold my child in my arms.

A few nights later, as I was preparing for bed, I went to the bedroom windows to make sure they were locked. As I pulled the curtain back, I thought, *If you're out there, baby, give me a sign.* I looked up into the dark sky as I always do. I have loved the stars since childhood. This time I saw something I had never seen before. The moon was full, and there was a perfect circle around it, which I'd seen before; but what made this night different was that the circle took up about half of the sky. I called my husband to look at it. He agreed that it was something he had never seen or heard of before either. It stayed like that for about half an hour and then faded.

We had decided to name the baby Isobella because I had a feeling the baby was a girl. For the next two months, either my husband or I saw or heard her name every day. Some would say that we were looking for it and that's why we noticed it. I disagree. It isn't the most common name, but it was showing up everywhere. My husband is not the kind just to go along with strange coincidences; he is a very grounded man. He knew something was going on. Slowly, we stopped seeing her name, not because we were adjusting to her being gone, but for some reason her name just wasn't there anymore. I was still very upset about her loss and cried for at least a year, and still do at times.

She had been due on May 17, and I was dreading that day coming. I cried more and more as the day approached. For some reason, on that day I actually forgot. I was at a store looking in the book section and came across a book with the title *Isobella*. I instantly remembered that it was her due date. I went home sad but happy at the same time. I had not felt her presence in months, but I knew she had come by to see me on the day she was meant to be born. I told my husband that I saw her name at the store, and he was surprised since he had seen it, too, on the side of a bus. I have seen her name occasionally since then but never daily as in the first two months after I lost her. I no longer feel that she is around us. I feel she has moved on. I am not a religious person at all; I am atheist. I do believe, however, that there is some sort of life after death, and my baby is now a part of that life. I miss my baby, and it hurts to know that she would be eighteen months old now. I feel an emptiness, a void.

I never know when something will remind me of my loss and the tears will flow. I have been initiated into a group of women who have experienced miscarriages, and I am now more sensitive to the loss of others. Before, I could offer condolences but had no real understanding.

I bought a tiny pair of gold shoes that I wear as a necklace, a reminder of the baby. My heart goes out to all the mothers who have lost a baby and to all of those who will.

Now living in California, Mutsumi was born and lived in Japan until the age of twenty-four. She wrote about her baby girls, Chie and Ai, and we began corresponding by e-mail.

Mutsumi and Babies Chie and Ai

I've lost two babies in the past. My first loss was about eighteen years ago, by abortion. My second loss was just two years ago, by miscarriage. I don't know whether they were boys or girls, but I somehow feel they were both girls. Since then, I've been hoping to see them in a dream, though it hasn't happened. My late brother had visited me in a dream a couple times, so I knew it was possible.

My encounter happened just a few months ago. I was walking my dog at the beach and looking at a young couple with a little child, about three years old, walking hand in hand. They seemed very happy. I thought about my lost babies and pictured myself walking with my two beautiful children hand in hand. Then all of a sudden, I saw two butterflies suddenly appear from nowhere and fly around me. They stayed with me for a while. It was beautiful. I felt warm and thought my babies were showing appreciation that I still think of them a lot.

I recently met with a woman who is my grief counselor with hospice. She is a very spiritual person and put all the pieces together for me so that I am finally able to see the light. I still don't know the exact reason why I have lost my two babies, though I know now that it is part of the big plan for me to grow spiritually.

I am planning to have a little ritual for my babies on Valentine's Day. I never thought I could let go of my sorrow, but I am ready now.

Mutsumi and I continued corresponding. At one point, I received three e-mails from her in one day and assumed she had mistakenly sent the same e-mail three times since the first two were identical. Just before deleting the third e-mail, I thought I should check it to be certain. Thankfully I did, because it contained another important message for me that read, "Once you start to move in the direction *they* want you to, you will find lots of information and the people you need." I wrote back to Mutsumi, thanking her for her message of support, but was surprised when she told me she hadn't written the message, and in fact it wasn't in her computer. I felt I was being guided to continue my research and receiving a reminder that I am not alone. Next, Mutsumi told me about another experience she had.

At age twenty-one, I had my first spiritual experience in connection with the abortion. I was four weeks pregnant, and my then-boyfriend was about to go to the United States for his studies. I was afraid and confused. After the anesthesia was induced, I went into a deep sleep. Suddenly, I saw a tremendous orange-reddish sphere rotating very fast in front of me. It somehow reminded me of a big mandala. The next thing I remember is that I was inside of it, in a whole different dimension. I felt I was part of the universe, and at the same time I was the universe itself. Time seemed altered. A blink of time seemed like eternity. I felt I became enormous, and at the same time it was as if I were microscopic. It was a very real sensation. Then, somehow, I was looking down on the Earth and saw all my worries, and I knew these concerns were nothing compared to this extraordinary experience. I still remember the peaceful and warm feeling I had; it was love.

I didn't talk about the abortion or my strange experience for some time. Even though the vision changed the way I look at life, I still suffered guilt and sadness for a very long time. I think I was depressed, and before I was able to let go of my grief, my second loss hit me.

I gave my babies Japanese names. The first is Chie, which means wisdom, because she gave me the wisdom of the universe. The second is Ai, and as you can imagine, it means love. She gave me the love that I'd needed for a long time.

Weeks later, Mutsumi wrote to me again about seeing one of her babies in a dream and about the good-bye ritual she and her husband performed.

Today is a very special day for me because I finally saw my second baby, Ai, in a dream. Actually, I had four similar dreams last night, all involving babies who were sick. I was in a hospice and saw another building next door, with many rooms and wooden doors. I was with a male doctor, who led me to one of the doors. I went in and saw a small crib filled with three or four babies that looked newly born. The doctor went to take care of the babies. I knew they were going to die, and I asked myself why they had to die.

At the end of the final dream, I saw a little girl about eighteen months old, the same little girl I had seen in one of the previous dreams. I heard a nurse saying I wasn't supposed to be there, but I went in the room anyway. I knelt down in front of the little girl and looked at her. She had beautiful, soft, curly brown hair that cascaded down over one of her eyes. She looked up at me, and I saw her beautiful brown eye (only one eye because her hair covered the other). She looked into my eyes. We looked at each other for a long time. Her eye was smiling, and it was the most beautiful eye I've ever seen. I woke up crying. It was a beautiful sunny morning, and I heard a bird singing and saw a bright light coming through the window. I felt warm and comforted. I realized then that it was my baby I had seen. It was a bittersweet feeling because I was so happy she had finally come to see me, but at the same time I was very sad because I missed her so much.

That morning, my husband and I went to the pier to do a good-bye ritual. We brought two white roses and said a prayer, and then put the flowers in the ocean. It took a long eighteen years for me to be able to finally let go of my grief. The amazing thing was we enjoyed it so much, without feeling sad or lonely. I feel very light now.

Thank you for the opportunity to tell my story. It is so nice that someone is really hearing what I'm saying, because I am having a hard time talking with many of my friends about what I'm going through. I guess that's why you need to write your book.

Life Goes On

I have tried to show throughout this brief study that communication is not merely possible with souls yet unborn to us, but that it is, in fact, happening with many mothers, fathers, other family members, and friends. Hearing from the other side in whatever form it might take is no longer farfetched or even unique. Too many people have made such contacts for all of them to be called crazy, and each experience seems to confirm another, while resonating deeply within each individual.

When I'd nearly finished writing the book, Tim, Kylie, and I attended Meghan's school Christmas choral recital. It had been an especially tiring day, both emotionally and physically, and I welcomed the opportunity to sit and relax without any demands. As we waited for the program to begin, I began to feel melancholy that it would be the last recital we'd attend at the elementary school since Meghan was in fifth grade and would be attending middle school the following year. In my mind, I reviewed the nine years of recitals we'd watched with Kylie and Meghan on stage, and I realized a chapter of my life was closing. I wanted to notice and appreciate every moment of the performance so that it would be ingrained in my memory.

Ninety third-graders walked up the steps of the stage and took their assigned positions. I searched the crowd of children for a face I might recognize before realizing I no longer knew a third-grader. Once the children were in place, the music teacher began calling out specific children's names to come forward to pick up their instruments and stand at the front of the stage. One by one, the children came forward, taking their places in the spotlight. I was briefly lost in thought until the last child's name was called.

"Dillon," the teacher called out. I sat up straight in the chair and looked to the stage to see what the little boy looked like. There was no movement among the children on stage. "Dillon?" she called out again as she looked anxiously through the sea of children's faces for his. Dillon didn't step forward. The children on stage and the multitude of parents in the audience were now eager for the missing child to appear so the performance could begin. The children began frantically looking among themselves for Dillon as the audience looked with curiosity and amusement for the lost little boy.

As though the star of the show were missing, the teacher called out nervously and with a hint of exasperation, "Where's Dillon?"

I smiled as the answer was softly whispered in my mind, "He's right here. He's right *here!*" A deep sigh of relief from the audience could be heard as Dillon emerged from the back row of children, seemingly oblivious to what the fuss was all about. My smile broadened as I got a glimpse of him. "Of course," I whispered to myself. He was a blonde-haired boy who wore an impish grin.

When signs of souls on the other side were close to me but too big for my mind to absorb or deal with, I questioned their authenticity. I pushed them away. Although I was being jolted awake, I'd been programmed not to believe. I realized that often the very phenomena I need to explore are the ones that challenge my belief system.

When I first began to experience communication with Dillon, I questioned at times whether I'd gone mad. Communication with him continued, however, whether it was through my auditory sense or received through meditation, self-hypnosis, psychics, coincidences, or simply sensing his presence. The skeptic in me attempted to find an explanation that was more plausible than what had actually happened, until my last wall of denial was crumbled when I asked for and received proof with the antique key. I found, too, that the experiences of those who contributed to this book have validated my own, and they might do the same for others who've kept their children's communication close to their hearts or were afraid to share such experiences openly.

For years, Dillon's loss felt only tragic, but now I see the gift he has given me as it continues to unfold in my life—a gift of spirit and soul, of knowing with certainty on a deep level that life is continuous. The soul lives on. I now recognize his gift was far greater than even the vision in the park that somehow instantly healed my relationship with my father. I understand it was Dillon's choice, his sacrifice, not to come for my greater good and that I must share this gift to help others.

My spiritual journey and growth began with his loss. Perhaps I even entered this life with such a plan but with free will to decide whether I'd make the choice that offered spiritual growth. All I know is that I am grateful I found the courage to break through barriers of doubt and fear to explore the spiritual path. Understanding and inner peace come only from the search, from spiritual awakening. Dillon's brief life made that possible, and for that I humbly and profoundly thank him for coming.

Even though we may believe in the continuity of life and that our loved ones are close to us in spirit, grieving and the pain of loss cannot be avoided. It is human and necessary to mourn our losses. When I first lost Dillon, I was in deep, numbing grief, but I no longer carry that sorrow. I think of him now only with love and gratitude that he came, if only for a brief moment of time. I take comfort in knowing more than ever before that my loved ones are still watching over me and remain strongly bonded to me through love. I am not alone. I never was. None of us are alone. Our loved ones surround us and are there for our celebrations and tragedies in life. And sometimes, when I least expect it, Dillon reminds me, "They're here. They're right *here!*"

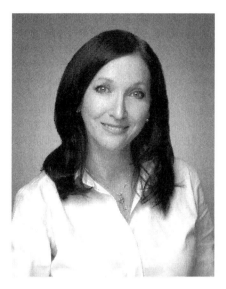

About the Author

Patricia lives with her husband Tim, daughters Kylie and Meghan in Tarpon Springs, Florida. She is a certified hypnotist in private practice, specializing both in helping parents connect with their lost children and in past-life regression. She has established a new field of research in communication with early loss babies, which is ongoing.

If you've had a communication experience with a lost baby and would like to share it with her, please write with as many details of your experience as possible, including how you feel as a result of the contact.

Angelbabies10527@aol.com

www.patriciamcgivern.com

Patricia is available to present lectures and workshops about her ongoing research in spirit communication with miscarried and other lost babies, as well as past lives. Contact her through her Web site to arrange speaking engagements or to check her upcoming travel schedule. If you would like to set up an appointment for a private session, you may also contact her by e-mail or through her Web site.

Additional copies of *Angel Babies: Messages from Miscarried and Other Lost Babies* can be purchased from www.Amazon.com, www.BarnesandNoble.com, www.Borders.com, www.BooksaMillion.com, or from www.iUniverse.com. Any bookstore may order copies from the publisher http://www.iUniverse.com, or from its distributors, Ingram Book and Baker & Taylor, or Chapters/Indigo in Canada.

Spiritual Advisers

Yvonne M. Gangone, C.Ht., PL.T.
Spiritual Medium
New York
(845) 469-8497
gift12@optonline.net

Maryanne Lane
freedommotion@yahoo.com

Don McIntosh
Astrologer and Spiritual Counselor
4105 Ocean Beach Blvd. #122
Cocoa Beach, Florida 32931

Christine Riley
Psychic Intuitive
(727) 447-8611
Clearwater, Florida
Noitall@tampabay.rr.com

Gail Rhoads
Clairvoyant
(352) 372-8039
4130 NW Thirteenth Street, Suite 204
Gainesville, Florida 32609

John Rogers
Professional Medium
Author, *The Medium Within*
(321) 733-1555
Melbourne, Florida
JRogers47@cfl.rr.com

Support Groups

George Anderson Support Groups
Andrew Barone, Director of George Anderson Grief Support
Programs
http://www.georgeanderson.com
Group or private sessions available.

The Compassionate Friends
P.O. Box 3696, Oak Brook, Illinois 6052203696
(630) 990-0010 or (877) 969-0010
http://www.compassionatefriends.org
A worldwide organization offering friendship, understanding, and support for bereaved parents, siblings, and grandparents.

Hospice
228 Seventh Street SE, Washington, DC 20003
(202) 546-4749
http://www.hospice-america.org
A care-giving team of professionals and volunteers working together to serve terminally ill patients and their families. Additionally, they provide support to those who've lost a member of their families, including babies.

M.I.S.S. Foundation
P.O. Box 5333, Peoria, AZ 85385
(623) 979-1000
http://www.missfoundation.org
An international organization providing immediate and ongoing support to grieving families.

Share Pregnancy and Infant Loss Support
National Share office, St. Joseph Health Center,
300 First Capitol Drive, St. Charles, Missouri 63301
Phone: (800) 821-6819   Fax (636) 947-7486
http://www.nationalshareoffice.com
For families bereaved by miscarriage, stillbirth, or neonatal death.

Pregnancy and Infant Loss Awareness Day is October 15. Light a
candle at 7:00 PM.
Join others who are doing the same throughout the world.

RELATED BOOKS AND WEB SITES

Life After Life by Raymond Moody, MD, PhD. http://www.RaymondMoody.com

Born To Live and *The Physician Within You* by Gladys T. McGarey, MD, MD(H). http://www.mcgareyfoundation.com

Our Children Forever: George Anderson's Messages from Children on the Other Side by Joel Martin and Patricia Romanowski, and *Lessons from the Light* by George Anderson and Andrew Barone. http://www.georgeanderson.com

Hello from Heaven by Bill Guggenheim and Judy Guggenheim. http://www.after-death.com

Stories of the Unborn Soul and *Soul Trek* by Elisabeth Hallet. http://www.light-hearts.com

Children's Past Lives and *Return from Heaven* by Carol Bowman, MS. http://www.childpastlives.org.

Made in the USA
San Bernardino, CA
15 March 2019